THE SCIENTIFIC MENOPAUSE HANDBOOK & GUIDE

A RESEARCH-BASED HANDBOOK ON HORMONES, PHYSICAL & MENTAL HEALTH, DIET AND EXERCISING

CARINA DAVENPORT

CONTENTS

INTRODUCTION

O ne minute, you are full of energy, and you know exactly what your body will do from one week to the next. Then, suddenly, you are struggling to get through the day without a few extra cups of coffee or an afternoon nap, you start removing your sweater even when it's freezing outside, and you have no idea how you will react to something that irritates you.

You're going through "the change". It happens to all women, usually after forty, but it may be sooner or later. It could occur suddenly for medical reasons, but it is usually a gradual change as your hormone levels become less predictable.

The hormones that have made your body what it is and do what it does since puberty are running amok. Up until now, they have naturally risen and fallen depending on where you are in your menstrual cycle, preparing your uterus to welcome a fertilized egg and support a pregnancy or, should conception not occur, cleaning it out for the next cycle.

If you were a textbook case, you would have been able to rely on this monthly cycle, knowing when you would have more energy than usual and when you would be a bit irritable. Now, everything has changed. Your cycle may be less than the average 28 days, or it could be much longer. You may even skip a period or two.

Along with the changes to your cycle, you may start experiencing other symptoms that show your reproductive hormones are misbehaving. Hot flushes, mood swings, and lack of libido, along with new health challenges such as high cholesterol and hypertension, become the new normal, leaving you wondering where you went wrong.

It may come as a surprise to you, especially if the women in your life are too embarrassed to talk about menopause. Sadly, millions of women enter this transitional stage of their lives with very little information, feeling like they have no one to turn to and ask about what is happening to their bodies. It makes it impossible to plan for and ensure you do everything you can to make the change in how your body works a blessing instead of a curse.

Knowledge about your reproductive hormones and their impact throughout your body, not only on your reproductive system, empowers you to take charge of your health and the rest of your life. It enables you to have meaningful conversations with your healthcare provider and make informed decisions about managing your fluctuating hormones and the consequences of hormonal changes in your body.

The answers you are looking for can be found in the chapters of this book. You will learn about the different stages of menopause and how your body gives clues about what is happening. There will be no more guessing about whether you are premenopausal, going through perimenopause, or already in menopause. This alone gives you a stepping stone to finding the best way to manage the transition.

You will discover that although most women go through natural menopause in their late forties and early fifties, there are other reasons your hormone levels change. For example, the surgical removal of your ovaries or some medication may alter them and suddenly cause menopause symptoms.

Of course, your armor would be incomplete if you are left unaware of the impact your changing hormones have on all parts and systems of your body. You are probably aware that you may experience changes in your metabolism, resulting in weight gain, but did you know such changes may also cause higher blood sugar and cholesterol levels? In addition, your cardiovascular system relies on estrogen and progesterone to function properly and maintain a normal blood pressure, and your bones need the hormones to remain strong and healthy.

When faced with the unavoidable and significant changes associated with the middle years of your life, you may want to run and hide, but with the focus on women's health in the healthcare industry, you now have more options for menopause management than the women who came before you.

Both women and their doctors are more aware of how critical it is for women's well-being to address hormonal fluctuations. Whether you choose hormone replacement therapy (HRT) or opt for nutritional supplements and natural therapies, you can continue to live a vibrant life and feel comfortable in your skin.

While your body may need a boost from medication and supplements, your lifestyle choices are crucial to a happy midlife transition. As such, what you choose to eat every day not only ensures you maintain your weight but also helps to prevent and manage any lifestyle-related health conditions that may crop up, like high blood pressure and diabetes.

Hence, a large portion of this guide explains the pros and cons of various diets for menopausal women. Beginning with a balanced diet and moving on to explore other popular eating styles, you will be able to pick the best diet for you to manage the symptoms you experience.

There is no such thing as a single best diet for everyone. Since menopause is associated with higher levels of inflammation, you may benefit from an omega-3, plant-rich Mediterranean diet, or if your blood sugar levels indicate that you are developing diabetes, a ketogenic diet might be better.

Your food choices are just one of the pillars of a healthy life stage change. Making regular physical activity that incorporates cardiovascular exercise, resistance training, and stretching for flexibility is good for both your body and your mind.

The final pillar is self-care. Some things about menopause can't be changed, but by being kind to yourself and making time for gratitude and mindfulness, your journey through the upheaval created by hormone changes can be smoother. Thus, learning to love yourself and accepting your changing body is a powerful tool in menopause management.

Until "the change", many women have put others' well-being before their own. Despite the annoying and sometimes debilitating symptoms, women must endure during menopause, it can be a time of self-discovery and self-love, opening the path for you to thrive and live your best life in your later years.

FROM PUBERTY TO MENOPAUSE

M enopause is a natural stage of a woman's life, yet it is so often talked about in hushed tones as if it is a taboo topic that is too embarrassing to be openly discussed. For this reason, it is a mystery for many women and is approached with a sense of dread. Moreover, in many societies, the midlife change is viewed negatively, with many believing it signifies the end of a woman's vitality.

It's time to set the record straight and learn to embrace the inevitable change associated with the middle years of your life. You may no longer be able to have babies, but does that mean you are not still useful and valued in your community?

There is a lesson to be learned by modern Western women from several traditional cultures scattered around the world who embrace women in their middle years. For one thing, women living in such cultures earn greater respect from their communities and take on new roles, such as herbal healers. Others are given "wise woman status", recognizing their life experiences and the value they add to society (Hall et al., 2007).

That's not to say midlife is not a challenge for these women. They also experience the same range of physical and mental symptoms and health-related issues as all women do. However, they are better prepared and are celebrated for their maternal wisdom.

No matter where you are, being a woman is complicated. Your community has different expectations of you depending on your stage of life, which is characterized by the changes occurring in your body. From childhood to puberty, from adolescence to adulthood, and from midlife to old age, your body rises to the challenge and adapts as your role in society shifts.

Menopause is shrouded in mystery. It is a complex process, and to make it even more confusing, every woman experiences it differently. It has had women and their healthcare providers flummoxed for centuries.

The best way to approach this important life change is to arm yourself with an in-depth knowledge of menopause and the possible effects it may have on how your body works. After all, as the saying goes, "forewarned is forearmed". In other words, if you know what you're up against when your hormone levels start fluctuating, you can put strategies in place to help you manage the transition and turn menopause into a positive life experience.

In this chapter, we explore menopause to dismiss the myths and misconceptions and reveal the positive aspects of becoming a wise woman. The physiological changes your body undergoes when your reproductive hormone levels start changing will also be unraveled. You will learn how to identify which stage of menopause you are experiencing.

This is the first step on your journey towards embracing your inner wisdom and becoming a powerful menopausal woman.

Hormonal Changes in Puberty

Before defining menopause, let's go back to the first reproductive transition you experienced as you changed from a girl to a woman - puberty. It signifies the beginning of your fertility and is characterized by a steep rise in several hormones that transform a girl's body into its adult form and makes it possible to conceive and support the growth of a baby.

What are hormones?

Are you ready for a quick physiology lesson? This section is full of big c0mplicated words, but persevere because it forms the foundation for understanding what is happening in your body.

To begin with, hormones are a crucial part of the endocrine system, which comprises several glands and organs throughout the body. These crucial physiological structures include the thyroid gland, adrenal glands, the pituitary gland, as well as the ovaries and testes. They make and release hormones that regulate all biological processes, including growth, maturation, metabolism, sexual function, mood, and even sleep. Hormones act as messengers to regulate the structure and function of the human body (Hormones | Endocrine Glands | MedlinePlus, n.d.).

When puberty begins in girls, and throughout their fertile years, gonadotropin-releasing hormone is released by the hypothalamus, a small but critical brain region. Its job is to stimulate the anterior pituitary gland to synthesize

follicle-stimulating hormone and luteinizing hormone (Casteel, n.d.), both of
which have an impact on the female reproductive system as described below:

1. **Follicle-stimulating hormone (FSH)** stimulates the growth of ovarian
   follicles. Girls are born with several hundred thousand of these fluid-filled sacs in their ovaries. At the beginning of each menstrual cycle,
   a few follicles begin to mature. Each contains an immature egg, but
   only one reaches maturity and is released into the fallopian tube to be
   fertilized. Follicles are crucial for female reproduction as they produce
   estrogen, one of the most important female sex hormones (Orlowski,
   n.d.).

2. **Luteinizing hormone (LH)** triggers ovulation. In addition, it stimulates the follicles to transform into the corpus luteum once the egg has
   been released in the middle of your menstrual cycle when you ovulate.
   It is a temporary organ that produces progesterone, another prominent
   female hormone that prepares the uterus for pregnancy (Nedresky, n.d
   .).

Estrogen and progesterone are not only critical for coordinating your menstrual
cycle. They also influence the structure and function of the female body.

There are numerous effects of **estrogen** on the body (Delgado, n.d.).

It helps with the development of breast tissues. Estrogen regulates the menstrual
cycle by promoting the thickening of the uterine lining in preparation for possible
pregnancy. Increased estrogen levels are associated with a shift in the distribution
of fat in the female body, leading to girls developing wider hips and a curvier
figure. Higher levels of estrogen promote the maturation of the pelvic bones
in preparation for childbirth. Estrogen contributes to the growth spurt girls
experience in adolescence by stimulating the growth plates in the long bones. The
maturation of the fallopian tubes, uterus, and cervix is dependent on rising levels
of estrogen in a girl's body.

While estrogen is the key driver of puberty, **progesterone**, which is produced
in the second half of the menstrual cycle, plays an equally important supporting
role. It has two crucial functions (Cable, n.d.):

1. Progesterone ensures the continued thickening and maintenance of the
   uterine lining after ovulation to support a potential pregnancy.

2. Progesterone contributes to the full development of the mammary
   glands and ducts in the breasts, preparing them for lactation.

Furthermore, the reproductive system isn't the only part of the body affected by
your sex hormones. They also influence a girl's mental health, metabolism, heart
health, and immune system.

Pre-Menopause: Your Fertile Years

Puberty sets the stage for your fertile years. Every month for three to four decades, several follicles begin maturing, with only one producing an egg that can be fertilized. Consequently, the number of follicles in your ovaries slowly begins to decline. The average woman will continue to have a regular menstrual cycle every 28 days (give or take a few days) from the age of 12 or 13 years until there are no more follicles left in her ovaries.

During this fertile stage of your life, there is a predictable fluctuation in estrogen and progesterone throughout the month, making it possible to get pregnant and support a healthy pregnancy. Both biological messengers have been shown to have several benefits for women's health over and above sexual function and fertility.

The health benefits of **estrogen** include (Patel et al., 2018):

Estrogen is involved in metabolism and maintaining healthy blood sugar levels. The immune system relies on estrogen to work properly by suppressing the inflammatory response. Estrogen supports the cells on your bones called osteoblasts, which handle the production of new bone tissue. Thus, the hormone is essential for bone health. The incidence of heart disease in women is much lower before menopause than after. One of the reasons is that estrogen helps to keep cholesterol levels under control. Estrogen has several effects on the central nervous system. It increases blood flow in the brain, reduces inflammation, and enhances the transfer of messages between nerve cells.

The health benefits of **progesterone** include (Nagy et al., 2021):

Progesterone helps to maintain the balance of salt and water in the body, which is crucial for regulating your blood pressure. The hormone is involved in the production of serotonin, a neurotransmitter that helps pass messages between the nerves in your brain. It is involved in controlling your mood, as well as your brain's ability to learn and remember things. It also plays a role in regulating your body temperature, your sleep patterns, your appetite, and your sexual behavior. During your fertile years, progesterone modulates your stress response by controlling the production of stress hormones such as cortisol. Progesterone protects women from various cancers, including uterine and colon cancer. By controlling your inflammatory response and the activation of your immune system, progesterone helps to boost your immunity.

Mid-Life Changes

After two to three decades of having predictable levels of these biological messengers at each stage of your menstrual cycle, it is not surprising women feel the effects of declining or fluctuating amounts of estrogen and progesterone in the body as they enter the second significant reproductive transition in their life cycle - menopause (Hoyt & Falconi, 2015).

For most women, menopause is a gradual transition from fertility to no longer being able to conceive and support a pregnancy. It is more like a slow dimming of a light than instantly flicking off a switch and is associated with several signs and symptoms that gradually creep up on you.

Menopause signifies the end of your reproductive years. With declining estrogen levels, your menstrual cycle becomes less predictable until it eventually stops altogether. When you have gone twelve months without having a period you are in menopause. However, there is a transition period of several years between fertility and menopause. Below is an outline of the stages of this midlife change.

Stages of menopause

There are three distinct stages of menopause, each characterized by a set of symptoms. Not all women experience the same sequence of events or signs and symptoms as their hormone levels change. It can make defining where you are in the journey challenging and frustrating. Some women will experience all the symptoms, from hot flashes to painful sex and sleepless nights, while others might breeze through the change, barely having noticed the transition. Let's look at each stage of menopause, starting with perimenopause, moving on to menopause, and ending in post-menopause.

Perimenopause

The journey usually begins with perimenopause in your mid to late forties or early fifties. It is a natural rite of passage for all women. It is as inevitable as having your first period in puberty. As such, it cannot be avoided, and being prepared for it empowers you to approach the midlife change with a plan for managing it to support your physical and mental health.

The result of lower levels of estrogen is a range of symptoms, including those listed below (Santoro, 2016):

- **Hot flashes** affect most women during perimenopause. If you have never experienced one, a hot flash is a sudden, intense heat experienced on the chest, neck, and face because of an overly reactive body thermostat caused by declining estrogen levels. They can also be accompanied by profuse sweating.

- **Poor sleep** becomes a problem for many women during this phase of their lives. It may be caused by night sweats (hot flashes while you are sleeping), or you may suddenly find it difficult to fall asleep and stay asleep.

- **Depressed mood** may become a problem for many women for the first time during perimenopause.

- **Anxiety levels** increase during menopause, even in women who haven't struggled with anxiety before.

- **Irregular menstrual cycles** become the norm. The closer you get to menopause, the longer the gap between your periods becomes. Initially, you may occasionally skip a period, but as you progress through your journey, you may experience gaps of 2 to 11 months between menstruation.

- **Vaginal dryness** is a symptom of perimenopause experienced by a third to a quarter of women because of low estrogen levels. It can cause itching, irritation, and discomfort.

- **Painful Sex** is another side effect of vaginal dryness, contributing to a drop in women's desire for sex.

- **Brain fog** is a common symptom of perimenopause. Think about how often you have walked into a room only to have forgotten what you had gone there for or looked for your glasses when wearing them. Jokes aside, brain fog can interfere with your daily productivity.

- **Fatigue** also makes it challenging to get through the day. Perimenopausal women may experience bouts of extreme fatigue.

- **Weight gain**, especially around your belly, creeps up on you in your forties. It often happens even though you have not changed anything in your diet or exercise routine.

The perimenopausal years are riddled with frustrating symptoms that sometimes seem to come out of the blue. One minute you are calm and loving life, the next, you are a raging lunatic, irritated by everything and everyone. "Meno rage" is real! So is crying at the drop of a hat. Those heart-wrenching television commercials will have you reaching for the tissue box whenever you see them.

Life goes on despite the mood swings and hot flashes. Somehow, it would be best if you could embrace this significant life change through a combination of diet, exercise, mindfulness, herbal remedies, and hormone replacement therapy. You know your body better than anyone else, so use your wisdom to discuss your options with your healthcare provider.

Menopause

Since menopause is a time of transition, the symptoms associated with peri-menopause may continue after you are officially in menopause and have not menstruated for more than 12 months. However, there are some new symptoms to look out for after your periods have stopped, including the following (Jin, 2017; Zouboulis et al., 2022):

Hair thinning occurs due to changes in the hair follicles on your scalp. Your hair may also grow slower than it did before.

Skin changes are associated with menopause. You may notice that your skin is no longer as elastic as before, resulting in wrinkles and sagging. You may also experience dryness, itching, changes in skin pigmentation, and slower wound healing.

Urinary symptoms that occur during menopause include having to go to the toilet more often and a higher risk of urinary tract infections.

On the plus side, some women report having fewer headaches as they get closer to menopause (Pavlović, 2020). In addition, moods may become more stable, and other perimenopause symptoms may become more predictable.

Post-Menopause

Life changes again after your body has gone through the final stages of menopause. You are now in post-menopause. After all the hormonal upheaval of perimenopause and menopause, your body gains a new equilibrium. You will no longer have to deal with fluctuating hormone levels and the wide range of symptoms that go with them. However, while you may see the back of some of your symptoms, it must be noted that some might linger and become a permanent feature and have to be managed throughout the rest of your life.

How to Prepare for Menopause

Preparing for menopause involves a proactive approach to managing the physical and emotional changes during this midlife transition. Use the following tips to ensure your body and mind are in the best possible shape before fluctuating hormones turn your world upside down.

- **Educate yourself:** Learn about your reproductive hormones, the impact they have on your body, and what happens when their levels start fluctuating during perimenopause.

- **Regular exercise:** Don't wait for hot flashes and sleepless nights before getting into shape. A fitter body has a greater resilience for change than a lazy one.

- **Balanced diet:** Eat a healthy balanced diet that includes foods from all the food groups. Good nutrition has a key role to play in promoting physical and mental health.

- **Maintain a healthy weight:** Losing weight is an uphill battle for many women, even before their hormones take them on a roller coaster ride. Do your best to keep your weight within the healthy range so that weight gain is easier to manage in your forties and fifties.

- **Self-care:** Learn how to say no to others and take time to look after your own needs. It is not a selfish thing to do. After all, you can't pour from an empty cup.

- **Stress management:** Life is stressful, even more so in the middle years of your life when you must juggle work, growing children, and aging parents. Learning effective stress management techniques can help ease the menopausal transition.

- **Healthcare:** Develop a relationship with your healthcare provider before the first signs and symptoms of menopause rear their heads. It will be easier to talk to them about menopause if you feel comfortable with them.

- **Treatment:** Whether or not you consider menopause a condition that requires medical intervention, keep an open mind when it comes to your treatment options. The effective management of menopausal change typically involves a blend of lifestyle changes, natural remedies, and hormone replacement therapy.

As you transition into post-menopause, take a moment to reflect on the changes your body has undergone since the day you were born with several hundred thousand follicles. First, you made the transition from being a girl to becoming a woman, making it possible for you to fall pregnant, support a growing fetus in your uterus, and give birth. Now, the sun is setting on your child-baring days as your body journeys to menopause and beyond.

This new phase may not be welcomed by you or society, but it is inevitable. As such, being prepared for the changes your body will experience can help you navigate the transition more smoothly. Knowing what to expect, your management options, and who to talk to for advice gives you an advantage many women do not have. You know your miraculous body better than anyone else, and your physical and mental health are in your hands. Empower yourself to move forward with the wisdom you have earned through living your feminine life.

TYPES OF MENOPAUSE

M enopause is an inevitable phase in a woman's life. The transition from fertility to your final period is as natural as the sun setting every evening. The only variables are when it will happen and how it will happen. For most women, it is an in-built gradual process, but genetics and the treatment for specific medical conditions can result in a more abrupt drop in estrogen and progesterone.

With that in mind, let's explore the different types of menopause, ranging from the natural midlife transition in your late forties and early fifties to genetic reasons causing the early onset of menopausal symptoms and abrupt menopause as a result of medical interventions. This chapter removes the veil of furtive self-consciousness to shed light on the distinct types of menopause and the implications of each.

Natural Menopause

Now that her children are older and can care for themselves, 48-year-old Jenny has been looking forward to exploring new hobbies and taking exciting trips with her husband. She has always been an active, fun-loving person who loves spending time outdoors. Lately, though, Jenny is waking up at 2 am drenched in sweat and exhausted in the afternoon, finding it difficult to complete her daily tasks. On top of that, her moods are all over the place, and her husband is starting to make excuses to stay out of her way. It occurred to Jenny that she might be experiencing "the change," and she booked an appointment with her doctor, who confirmed that she was indeed in the throes of perimenopause.

While your symptoms may be different from Jenny's, her story paints a picture of natural menopause, the gradual process that unfolds as a woman enters the middle years of her life. It typically begins between 45 and 55 and lasts seven to 14 years.

The gradual reduction in the production of estrogen and progesterone in the ovaries causes natural menopause. Your menstrual cycle becomes erratic, and you must deal with the physiological consequences of fluctuating hormones as your body seems to develop a mind of its own. Hot flashes, night sweats, mood swings, and changes in sexual function become the order of the day as you approach your final menstrual period.

It is not surprising that emotional and psychological upsets often accompany natural menopause. After all, the body you've been living in for 30 years since puberty is changing, and generally not in a good way. The physical symptoms can leave you feeling depressed and anxious, wondering what life has in store for you as you age. You may experience a range of emotions, including a sense of loss, changes in self-esteem, and reflections on aging.

Fortunately, menopause is better understood than when your grandmother experienced the transition. It empowers you to prepare physically and mentally for the symptoms you are likely to experience and seek timely guidance from your healthcare practitioner to get you through it (What Is Menopause? | National Institute on Aging, n.d.).

Premature Menopause (<40 Years)

Lindsay has been a bit concerned about her health recently. She is a healthy, fairly fit 37-year-old mother of two teenage boys. Yet, she has been having heart palpitations, battling with a low mood, and cranking up the air conditioner at the office even when her colleagues are feeling cold. It has become a bit of a joke around the office. After discussing her symptoms with her mother, she learned that her mom started menopause at the age of 36. Lindsay felt a combination of relief and despair as she booked an appointment with her doctor, hoping to find a solution for her symptoms. After a few blood tests and a thorough assessment of Lindsay's health, her doctor confirmed that she was going through premature menopause and gave Lindsay a few suggestions for the management of her symptoms.

One percent of women are surprised by menopause symptoms before their 40th birthday. Like Lindsay, it can be caused by a genetic predisposition, especially if your mother or sisters also had to deal with premature menopause.

However, it can also be a consequence of an autoimmune disease like rheumatoid arthritis or thyroid disorders or due to the treatment of a medical condition such as cancer with radiation or chemotherapy. While such treatments are critical for managing and curing certain diseases, they can bring about significant challenges for women facing the abrupt onset of menopause as well as dealing with the physical and psychological consequences of the health condition.

Premature menopause poses a unique set of physical and emotional challenges. Women may grapple with issues related to fertility loss at an earlier age than expected, which may have an impact on family planning as well as their identity. In addition, the impact of the health risks associated with the decline in reproductive hormones, such as osteoporosis, heart disease, and diabetes, are greater. In other words, the earlier you start menopause, the more mindful you must be of your overall health (Okeke et al., 2013).

Menopause is a trying time for women who experience natural menopause in their late forties, but it can be even more challenging when it happens too soon. While you may not be prepared early in life, reach out to people who can help you. Consult with your healthcare provider for advice on treatment options and support for your mental well-being.

Early Menopause (Between 40 and 44 Years)

Karen is a career woman who spent her thirties proving herself as a successful attorney. She always dreamed of having a beautiful home with a loving husband and two adorable children. She had her first child when she was 38 and started trying for her second when she turned 40. After a few months, she skipped her period. When she took a pregnancy test, she was disappointed to discover that she was not pregnant. She decided to ask her doctor for advice. After a thorough assessment of Karen's health, her doctor informed her that it was highly unlikely that she would be able to conceive and carry a baby to term because she was in early menopause. Karen had been so busy keeping up with work and a busy toddler that she had passed off her other symptoms of early menopause, such as rising anxiety and mood swings, as a consequence of burning the candle at both ends.

The difference between early menopause and premature menopause is that early menopause occurs after the age of 40 and before the age of 45, within the expected age range of natural menopause. Research suggests that early menopause occurs in 5 to 10% of women, affecting their fertility and general physical and mental health.

While this still falls within the normal range of menopausal age, women experiencing early menopause may come up against some distinct challenges compared to those entering menopause later. One key aspect of early menopause is managing the potential overlap of midlife transitions. Many women in their early forties are moving up in their careers, their aging parents need more attention, and the dynamics of their own families are changing with their children getting ready to leave the nest. Navigating menopause alongside these life changes can intensify the overall impact on a woman's well-being (Peycheva et al., 2022).

Physiologically, women undergoing early menopause may experience symptoms like those in natural menopause, but the timing makes managing your body's transition more challenging. As a powerful, if younger, menopausal woman, it makes sense to seek help. Consider taking advice on getting emotional support, making practical adjustments to your lifestyle habits, and discussing potential medical interventions to help you manage the impact of your unique combination of symptoms to improve your overall quality of life during this transitional period.

Surgically Induced Menopause

Kate had suffered from painful, heavy menstrual periods from a young age. She was diagnosed with endometriosis in her twenties and treated with a combination of medication, supplements, and lifestyle changes. By the time she was 35, the condition had advanced, and first-line treatments were no longer effective. Her doctor advised Kate to have a hysterectomy to remove her uterus and both ovaries. Before making her decision, Kate discussed the consequences of the surgery with her doctor, who warned her that she would experience an abrupt menopausal transition as she would no longer have her ovaries to produce estrogen and progesterone. After careful consideration and a treatment plan in place, she went ahead with the surgery.

Surgically induced menopause is a distinct type that results from surgical interventions such as hysterectomy (removal of the uterus) and oophorectomy (removal of one or both ovaries). These procedures can be performed for several reasons, including treating gynecological conditions, such as fibroids, endometriosis, or advanced polycystic ovarian syndrome, or for prophylactic purposes, such as preventing ovarian cancer in genetically susceptible women.

Unlike natural or premature menopause, surgically induced menopause is abrupt, and women may experience more intense symptoms. Consequently, the sudden loss of hormonal production from the ovaries can lead to more severe hot flashes, mood swings, and other common menopausal symptoms. Additionally, women undergoing such surgeries may face emotional and psychological challenges caused by the sudden and irreversible end to their ability to get pregnant.

The implications of surgically induced menopause extend beyond symptom management. Research suggests that the ovaries should be preserved, if possible, in women younger than 45 years to reduce the health-related consequences of sudden early menopause. However, in women whose ovaries must be removed, hormone replacement therapy (HRT) is usually recommended to alleviate symptoms and reduce the risk of long-term chronic health conditions associated with the loss of estrogen production. However, the decision to pursue HRT is complex and should be tailored to the woman's unique medical history, risk factors, and personal preferences (Hickey et al., 2009).

Chemically or Medically Induced Menopause

Helen found a cancerous lump in her breast when she was 36 and had to have chemotherapy to treat it. After a few weeks of treatment, she started noticing that she was having hot flashes and she was struggling to think clearly. Even though her doctor had told her about the side effects of her treatment, it didn't occur to her that she was experiencing the beginning of her menopausal transition. However, the symptoms worsened as her cancer treatment progressed, and her ovaries stopped producing estrogen.

Chemically or medically induced menopause can be caused by cancer treatments like chemotherapy and radiation therapy, which can damage ovarian tissue, leading to a rapid decline in hormone production and a sudden appearance of intense menopause symptoms. Additionally, medications like gonadotropin-releasing hormone (GnRH) agonists, used to treat conditions such as endometriosis and uterine fibroids, can temporarily suppress ovarian function, mimicking menopause.

Chemically induced menopause shares similarities with natural menopause, including symptoms like hot flashes, mood changes, and vaginal dryness. However, in some cases, it is reversible, and ovarian function may return to normal after the completion of treatment.

Managing chemically induced menopause is a team effort. Physicians work closely with patients to address the specific concerns related to their medical condition and the impact of induced menopause on their overall well-being. Supportive care, including psychological counseling and lifestyle adjustments, is integral to helping women navigate this unexpected early transition to menopause (Purohit et al., 2019).

Holistic Understanding and Personalized Approaches

The journey through menopause is not a one-size-fits-all experience. Women familiar with the midlife transition may expect the first symptoms to appear in their late forties to early fifties, but many are surprised by the early arrival of *the change*. By recognizing and addressing the distinct aspects of natural, premature, early, surgically induced, and chemically induced menopause, we can pave the way for a more comprehensive and compassionate understanding of this transformative life stage.

HORMONAL CHANGES

The hormonal shifts that trigger the transition into menopause are a natural progression in a woman's life. Changing levels of these influential biological messengers have an impact on almost all parts and systems in the body, altering the way your body works. For this reason, understanding these hormonal changes is crucial for navigating the challenges and embracing the opportunities that go with this transformative stage in your life.

Overview of Hormonal Changes

Your ovaries have played a central role in your reproductive system since puberty. However, as the number of follicles drops, the less active the ovaries become. The hormonal changes that occur during menopause are caused by this natural decline in the normal functioning of your ovaries. Since they handle making and releasing the key reproductive hormones, estrogen, and progesterone, a reduction in their activity results in lower levels of these hormones throughout the body, ultimately resulting at the end of menstruation and fertility.

In addition to reduced production of estrogen and progesterone, levels of other hormones like follicle-stimulating hormone and testosterone are also altered during menopause. While lower levels of estrogen and progesterone are the primary cause of the range of symptoms experienced by women during the menopausal transition, the impact of the others cannot be ignored (Santoro & Randolph, 2011).

Let's continue our lesson in physiology from Chapter 1 and unravel the biological changes that signify your growth into your well-earned role as a wise matriarch.

Decline of estrogen and progesterone

Estrogen

As you learned in the first chapter, estrogen is produced by the follicles in the ovaries. However, when women are born, their ovaries are filled with hundreds of thousands of follicles, and no more are produced throughout their life. Consequently, the number of follicles you are born with acts as a limiting factor on your fertility. Their number falls with every menstrual cycle, and the closer you get to midlife, the less there is to produce adequate amounts of estrogen. The result... hot flashes, night sweats, and loss of libido (Santoro & Randolph, 2011).

Progesterone

You will remember that progesterone is produced in the second half of your menstrual cycle by the corpus luteum, the temporary organ formed by the follicles after ovulation. Since the number of follicles drops during the menopausal transition and you may start skipping periods, with your cycle shifting from 28-30 days to 60 or more days, progesterone production also declines. Although less research has focused on the impact of reduced progesterone levels, it is a critical aspect of the transition to menopause (Santoro & Randolph, 2011).

Follicle-stimulating hormone (FSH)

FSH was the first hormone discussed in Chapter 1. Without the release of FSH from the pituitary gland, the ovaries would not be stimulated to produce estrogen. These two biological messengers work together in a bidirectional feedback mechanism. In other words, when estrogen levels are low, the pituitary gland is stimulated to release FSH, and as they climb, less FSH is produced.

During menopause, when ovarian function becomes limited, estrogen levels drop, and as a result, FSH levels rise. Therefore, elevated FSH levels indicate that the body is trying to stimulate the ovaries to produce more estrogen. However, the ovaries' responsiveness to FSH diminishes as menopause progresses, leading to an overall decline in estrogen production. An increase in FSH levels is a key marker used in diagnosing menopause and understanding the hormonal dynamics at play during this phase.

Fluctuations of testosterone

Although often considered a male hormone, testosterone also plays a role in women's health, contributing to libido, energy levels, and overall vitality. The ovaries also produce it; therefore, during menopause, levels of this hormone decrease (Santoro & Randolph, 2011).

Impact of Fluctuating Hormones on Physical and Mental Health

Physical Health

The hormonal changes during menopause have far-reaching implications for women's physical health. The decline in estrogen and testosterone, for example, not only contributes to the common signs and symptoms of menopause but also increases the risk of cardiovascular disease, muscle loss, declining brain health, metabolic disorders, and bone-related issues.

Maintaining a healthy lifestyle becomes paramount during menopause to reduce these risks. Regular exercise, a balanced diet, and avoiding tobacco and excessive alcohol consumption can positively impact bone health, cardiovascular function, and overall well-being.

Impact on Mental Health

The hormonal changes during menopause also exert a significant influence on mental health. Fluctuations in estrogen levels are linked to mood swings, irritability, and an increased risk of depression and anxiety.

Cognitive changes, often referred to as *brain fog* or difficulty concentrating, are also common during menopause. The effects of hormonal fluctuations on the neurotransmitters and the brain cause these changes. Effective stress management techniques, regular physical activity, and a supportive social network are crucial components of managing the mental health aspects of menopause.

A combination of factors, including biological, psychological, and sociocultural aspects causes the impact of hormonal changes on mental health. Open communication with your healthcare provider, the support of friends and family, and access to mental health resources can all contribute to a more positive and resilient mental health journey through menopause.

IMPACT OF MENOPAUSE ON WOMEN'S HEALTH

A s if night sweats and extreme mood swings, among all the other irritating and sometimes debilitating symptoms of menopause, were not enough, the fluctuating levels of estrogen also affect your health. The results of routine blood tests show that your body is not as healthy as it once was, and you cannot help but notice that your pants are getting tighter.

As mentioned in the previous chapter, although changing levels of progesterone and testosterone also contribute to your new health issues, estrogen has the greatest impact throughout your body. Since it is involved in supporting your immune and nervous systems, as well as your metabolism and heart health, it protects you from chronic diseases. That is, until menopause. Then, it can seem like all hell breaks loose, and your doctor starts talking to you about high blood pressure and raised cholesterol levels. They suggest getting your bone mineral density checked, and it is time to start having regular mammograms. And what's with the weight gain? Why is it so difficult to lose weight?

You will find many of the answers to these problems in this chapter, covering the effects of menopause on your skin and bones, your heart health, and changes to your metabolism, which result in weight gain and a rise in blood cholesterol and sugar levels. The changes that occur in your vagina and bladder will also be discussed, as well as the link between menopause and an underactive thyroid.

Use the information provided here as a stepping stone towards having an informed discussion with your healthcare provider about your health and well-being during your menopausal transition and beyond. They can guide you and offer treatment and management advice tailored to your unique midlife requirements.

Skin and Bones: The External and Internal Support System

Your skin is not immune to the effects of menopause. Estrogen plays a vital role in supporting skin health. It is the body's largest organ, forming a barrier between your vital organs and the environment. As such, it reflects external health factors such as exposure to the sun and can also show signs of internal health issues.

During menopause, the drop in estrogen levels results in changes to the structure and function of the skin. The impact of declining estrogen levels on collagen production causes reduced skin elasticity and the appearance of wrinkles. In addition, lower estrogen levels affect how much oil your skin makes, potentially causing dry skin. Let's unravel the reasons behind aging skin in midlife.

Skin Changes

Collagen and Elasticity: The Building Blocks of Skin

Collagen is a protein that provides structural support to the skin. It is crucial for maintaining its firmness and elasticity. Estrogen stimulates collagen production, and as its levels decrease during menopause, the skin may lose some of its resilience. In other words, as the amount of collagen in the skin drops, the skin becomes thinner, and folds begin to appear, resulting in wrinkles, fine lines, and sagging skin. Not only is the skin's appearance affected by lower estrogen levels, but it can also take longer for wounds to heal (Lephart & Naftolin, 2022).

To counteract these effects, women can incorporate collagen-boosting ingredients, such as retinoids and peptides, into their skincare routine. In addition, collagen-containing skin preparations and oral supplements have also been shown to be beneficial for increasing collagen levels. These formulations can stimulate collagen production and promote healthier, more youthful-looking skin (Al-Atif, 2022).

Oil Production and Hydration: Striking the Right Balance

Dry, itchy skin is usually the first sign of skin aging because of a drop in estrogen levels. This is because the hormone not only affects the skin's structure but also influences sebum production, the skin's natural oil. As estrogen levels drop, so, less oil is produced by the sebaceous glands, affecting the skin's hydration. The result is drier skin, itching, flakiness, and a dull complexion.

To combat dry skin, women can use moisturizers that contain ingredients like hyaluronic acid, glycerin, and ceramides. These substances help retain moisture and create a protective barrier, preventing excessive water loss from the skin (Ryczkowska et al., 2022).

Sun Sensitivity: Guarding Against UV Rays

While the sun's UV rays are crucial to producing bone-health-promoting vitamin D, the decline in estrogen during the menopausal transition and beyond can make the skin more susceptible to sun damage. Estrogen has photoprotective effects, which help shield the skin from the harmful effects of ultraviolet (UV) radiation. As estrogen levels decrease, women may become more prone to sunburn and long-term sun damage, including age spots and uneven pigmentation.

Also, excessive exposure to the sun has been shown to intensify the impact of lower estrogen levels on collagen production. Therefore, not only does your skin become more susceptible to sun damage, but spending too much time in the sun without the proper skin protection can accelerate the formation of fine lines and wrinkles.

Hence, sunscreen becomes a crucial part of skincare during menopause. Women should use a broad-spectrum sunscreen with a high SPF, applying it generously to all exposed skin, even on cloudy days (Park et al., 2021).

Bone Health

As you know, beauty - and health - is not skin deep. Beneath the skin, menopause also has a significant impact on bone health. Estrogen plays a critical role in maintaining bone mineral density by regulating the activity of osteoblasts and osteoclasts, the cells responsible for building and breaking down bone tissue. Before menopause, these two types of cells work together to maintain the delicate balance of bone mineral density, ensuring that your bones are strong and healthy.

The drop in estrogen levels during midlife disrupts this balance, reducing the amount of bone tissue made and increasing the amount lost, thus contributing to accelerated bone loss and increasing the risk of osteoporosis and fractures. Here, we discuss the precautions to prioritize bone health when entering menopause.

Osteoporosis: The Silent Threat

Osteoporosis, characterized by weakened and porous bones, becomes a significant concern for menopausal women. Research suggests that 1 in 3 women over the age of 50 will suffer a bone fracture as a result of the metabolic bone disorder in their lifetime. Furthermore, once you have experienced a fracture, the chance of suffering another is extremely high. As such, preventive measures are critical to reduce the risk of fractures, particularly in the spine, hips, and wrists (Sozen et al., 2017).

Adequate intake of calcium and vitamin D, along with vitamin K, magnesium, and protein, is crucial for maintaining bone health. It is recommended that women should aim for 1,200 milligrams of calcium per day, either through dietary sources like dairy products and leafy greens or supplements if necessary. The main source of vitamin D, which facilitates calcium absorption, is sunlight exposure. There are very few foods that contain significant amounts of this micronutrient, making supplementation necessary, especially if you live in an area that does not receive a lot of sunlight. Refer to Chapter 7 for more details.

While nutrition is the cornerstone of bone health, weight-bearing exercises, such as walking, jogging, and resistance training, help stimulate bone formation and improve overall bone density. On the other hand, Yoga and Pilates focus on balance and flexibility, thus helping to reduce your risk of falls and fractures. Engaging in a regular exercise routine not only strengthens your bones but also supports your joint health and overall physical well-being. See Chapter 11 for some ideas on incorporating exercise into your daily routine.

Cardiovascular Health: Navigating the Heart's New Rhythms

Estrogen has cardioprotective effects, influencing cholesterol levels and promoting healthy blood vessel function. In other words, the reproductive hormone promotes heart health by keeping your cholesterol levels under control and preventing the buildup of fatty deposits in the arteries. The drop in estrogen levels during menopause, therefore, increases the risk of cardiovascular diseases such as heart disease and stroke. As a result, you must be mindful of maintaining a heart-healthy lifestyle that includes regular exercise, a balanced diet, and managing other cardiovascular risk factors like hypertension and high blood sugar levels, as outlined below.

Cholesterol Levels

Estrogen has a favorable impact on cholesterol levels, promoting higher levels of high-density lipoprotein (HDL or "good" cholesterol) and lower levels of low-density lipoprotein (LDL or "bad" cholesterol). This balance helps protect against atherosclerosis, a condition where plaque builds up in the arteries, causing blockages and restricting blood flow.

With estrogen levels decreasing during menopause, there is a shift in this balance, potentially leading to raised LDL cholesterol levels. Consequently, it would be best if you prioritized a heart-healthy diet, rich in fruits, vegetables, whole grains, and lean proteins and low in saturated fats and highly processed foods to help manage cholesterol levels (Ryczkowska et al., 2022).

Blood Vessel Function

Estrogen contributes to the proper functioning of the endothelium, the inner lining of blood vessels. It helps maintain the dilation and constriction, or the relaxation and contraction, of blood vessels, ensuring blood flows efficiently no matter whether you are relaxing with a good book or hiking with your family. As estrogen levels decline during menopause, the endothelium may become less responsive, contributing to increased arterial stiffness, which may cause a rise in blood pressure (Miller & Duckles, 2008).

Lifestyle modifications such as regular exercise, smoking cessation, and stress management can help support vascular function. These measures, along with a balanced diet described in Chapter Seven, promote overall cardiovascular health and reduce the risk of high blood pressure and related complications.

Responsive Cardiovascular System

Assuming you have a healthy heart, it has been beating with a regular rhythm since the day you were born. It works harder when you are stressed or exercising and slower when you are relaxing, but you have seldom been aware of it beating inside your chest. This may change as you enter the menopausal transition.

Estrogen is involved in how your cardiovascular system reacts to various stimuli. For this reason, as levels decrease during menopause, you may experience changes in your heart rate and the regulation of your blood pressure. This can cause heart palpitations and contribute to an increased risk of developing cardiovascular diseases, including heart attacks and strokes (Li et al., 2014).

Regular cardiovascular exercise, such as brisk walking, cycling, or swimming, helps maintain the health and efficiency of the cardiovascular system. Exercise strengthens the heart muscle, improves blood vessel function, and enhances cardiovascular fitness.

Weight Gain and Metabolism

Although the details of weight gain during menopause are discussed in detail in Chapter Eight, it must also be mentioned here. Changes in your metabolism that cause weight gain are a common and frustrating complication for many women during the middle years of their life. During perimenopause, your weight can increase by an average of one pound (½ kg) annually. Not only do you gain weight, but your muscle mass also drops, further impacting your metabolic rate as it is your lean muscle tissue that burns calories in your body.

Hormonal fluctuations can cause reduced insulin sensitivity, resulting in raised blood sugar levels and increased fat storage, especially around the organs of the abdomen. These changes increase the risk of developing metabolic syndrome and cardiovascular issues. Adopting a healthy diet and engaging in regular physical

activity promote health throughout your life, but they become even more critical during this phase of your life to manage weight and support overall well-being (Ranjan et al., 2019).

Impact on the Genitourinary System

Another part of your anatomy that has served you well up until now is your genitourinary system consisting of your vagina, urethra, and bladder. Menopause brings about changes to this personal part of your body, resulting in discomfort, itching, and an increased risk of urinary tract infections, symptoms that can affect your quality of life.

Vaginal Changes

Estrogen plays a crucial role in the structure and function of vaginal tissue. It supports blood flow, maintains the thickness and elasticity of the tissue, and helps keep the lining of the vagina moist. As estrogen levels decline, the vaginal lining may become thinner, drier, and less elastic—a condition known as vaginal atrophy. This can result in symptoms such as vaginal dryness, itching, burning, and pain and discomfort during intercourse.

Topical estrogen therapies, such as creams or vaginal rings, can be effective in addressing vaginal atrophy. These localized treatments provide a controlled release of estrogen to the vaginal tissue, promoting its health and relieving symptoms. Regular sexual activity or the use of a water-based lubricant during intercourse may also help alleviate discomfort (Bleibel, n.d.).

Urinary Symptoms

Menopause-related alterations to the tissue in the vagina cause changes to the vaginal microbiome. This is the name given to the colonies of bacteria that live in the vagina and urethra and contribute to keeping the tissues healthy by preventing vaginal and urinary tract infections. Consequently, as the environment in the vagina changes, the type and number of bacteria is also altered, increasing the risk of more frequent infections in both the vagina and the bladder. Staying hydrated, practicing good hygiene, and emptying the bladder regularly can reduce the risk of urinary tract infections (Bleibel, n.d.).

Another problematic and potentially embarrassing problem experienced by many women is "leaking" when they cough, sneeze, jump, or laugh too hard. This is a result of the weakening of the pelvic floor muscles that help to control your bladder. Weaker pelvic floor muscles because of general degeneration in the genitourinary system may lead to urinary incontinence or the involuntary leakage of urine.

Pelvic floor exercises, commonly known as Kegel exercises, can help strengthen the muscles that support the bladder and urethra. These exercises are easy to perform and can be incorporated into a daily routine to improve urinary control (López-Pérez et al., 2023).

Hot Flashes and Night Sweats: The Internal Furnace

As previously discussed, hot flashes and night sweats, collectively known as vasomotor symptoms, are hallmark features of menopause, affecting up to 74% of menopausal women and up to 88% of women during perimenopause. These sudden, intense sensations of heat and sweating can significantly affect a woman's daily life and sleep quality. Perhaps one of the most widely recognized symptoms of menopause, hot flashes, and night sweats are a result of hormonal fluctuations impacting the body's temperature regulation.

The exact cause of personal menopausal heat waves is not fully understood, but hormonal fluctuations, particularly the decline in estrogen, play a central role. The hypothalamus, the region of the brain that regulates body temperature, appears to be sensitive to changes in estrogen levels, leading to women feeling hot, even in response to minor temperature changes.

While hormone replacement therapy (HRT) can be effective in managing vasomotor symptoms, some women prefer non-hormonal approaches. Lifestyle modifications can be crucial in reducing the frequency and severity of hot flashes and night sweats (Rapkin, 2007). Refer to the next Chapter for more details on your treatment options.

Hypothyroidism: Navigating the Hormonal Crossroads

Menopause and hypothyroidism are two distinct medical conditions, but they can be linked in several ways. They share common symptoms, such as fatigue, weight gain, and mood changes, making it essential to differentiate between them. In addition, the drop in estrogen levels during menopause can sometimes influence thyroid function. Therefore, women experiencing symptoms of an underactive thyroid gland (hypothyroidism) should undergo thorough testing to determine the appropriate treatment, which may include thyroid hormone replacement therapy.

To understand this connection, it's essential to grasp the basic concepts of each condition.

Menopause: As you know, menopause is a natural biological process that marks the end of a woman's reproductive years. It typically occurs in the late forties to early fifties and is defined by the cessation of menstrual periods. During menopause, the ovaries gradually reduce the production of estrogen and progesterone, leading to various physical and hormonal changes.

Hypothyroidism: The thyroid gland is shaped like a butterfly and is found in the front of your neck. Consequently, hypothyroidism is a condition where the thyroid gland is underactive and does not produce enough thyroid hormones, primarily thyroxine (T4) and triiodothyronine (T3). These hormones regulate metabolism, energy levels, and overall body function. When thyroid hormone levels are low, it can result in a range of symptoms, including fatigue, weight gain, cold intolerance, mood disorders, joint and muscle pain, dry skin, hair loss, slow heart rate, irregular menstrual periods, and cognitive difficulties (*Hypothyroidism (Underactive Thyroid) - NIDDK*, 2022).

Link between Menopause and Hypothyroidism:

Hormonal Changes: Menopause and hypothyroidism both involve significant hormonal changes, albeit different hormones with different functions. However, the decline in estrogen during menopause can sometimes unmask or intensify underlying thyroid issues. In addition, changes in sex hormone levels can affect how the thyroid gland functions, resulting in a change in thyroid hormone levels.

Symptom Overlap: Most symptoms of hypothyroidism overlap with those of menopause, making it challenging to differentiate between the two conditions. For example, both may cause fatigue, mood changes, and weight gain. This similarity in symptoms can lead to a delay in the diagnosis of hypothyroidism in menopausal women.

Thyroid Function and Menopausal Hormone Replacement Therapy: Research suggests that menopausal hormone replacement therapy, which involves the use of estrogen and progesterone to manage menopausal symptoms, might influence the amount of thyroid hormones available in the blood in women who have pre-existing hypothyroidism. It is, therefore, important for women undergoing menopausal hormone replacement therapy to have their thyroid function monitored regularly (Thyroid and Menopause Article, n.d.).

Increased Risk in Postmenopausal Women: Some studies have suggested that the risk of hypothyroidism may increase in postmenopausal women. The exact mechanisms are not fully understood, but they're believed to involve complex interactions between hormonal changes and genetic predispositions (Gietka-Czernel, 2017).

Impact on Metabolism: Both menopause and hypothyroidism can affect metabolism. The decline in estrogen during menopause can contribute to changes in body composition, while hypothyroidism directly affects metabolic rate. The combination of these factors can sometimes lead to weight gain in postmenopausal women with hypothyroidism.

It's important for women experiencing symptoms related to menopause or hypothyroidism to seek medical advice. A thorough evaluation, including blood tests to assess thyroid function, can help differentiate between these conditions. Effective management often involves a combination of hormone replacement therapy, if necessary, and thyroid hormone supplementation. Regular monitoring and collaboration with healthcare professionals is crucial for optimal care.

Consult with Your Healthcare Provider

Menopause may be inevitable, but with growing awareness amongst women and their healthcare providers, it is no longer a taboo topic or something that must be endured. The changes in your hormone levels can make you sweat and itch. They can also have a profound impact on your health. With this in mind, it is crucial for your overall health and well-being to consult with your healthcare practitioner when you notice the signs and symptoms of menopause. They can offer you support and guide you in the best way to manage your health in the middle years of your life and beyond.

MENOPAUSE MANAGEMENT

*M*andy is in her late forties. She's been struggling to get enough sleep lately because she wakes up several times a night drenched in sweat. Some nights it is so bad she must change her pajamas and her bedsheets. Mandy is also having overwhelming mood swings; one minute, she is feeling happy and carefree, and the next thing she knows, she is hit with an explosive anger that has everyone around her running for cover. However, one of the biggest challenges Mandy is facing is a complete lack of interest in being intimate with her husband. Up until now, Mandy has ignored her symptoms, adamant that she is not going through the menopausal change. However, her symptoms have started affecting her quality of life, so she has decided to reach out to her doctor to find out what she can do to get back to being her old self.

You are not alone if you can relate to Mandy's story. In the past, it was common for women to keep quiet about what was happening in their bodies, ignoring all the unpleasant changes they were experiencing. Many modern women still feel ashamed to talk about "the change". Fortunately, progress is being made, and not only are women more open about their hot flashes and low libidos, but there are also many more options available to help manage their declining levels of reproductive hormones.

Whether you prefer to take advantage of the advances in modern medicine or feel more comfortable with nutritional supplements and herbal remedies, there is an effective solution to help you through menopausal change with fewer symptoms and better health. These options are outlined in this chapter, empowering you to have an informed conversation about your well-being with your healthcare provider.

Hormone Replacement Therapy

Hormone Replacement Therapy (HRT) is a medical intervention designed to alleviate the symptoms of menopause and prevent the onset of health conditions like osteoporosis associated with declining hormone levels. Like the birth control pill, HRT is taken to adjust your hormone levels and includes a combination of estrogen and progesterone in various forms to imitate the hormones produced by your ovaries.

Estrogen occurs naturally in several forms, including estriol and estradiol. Some HRT formulations include the hormone in one of these forms. Others use conjugated equine (horse) estrogen, which is reportedly the most prescribed form of estrogen in the U.S. Although their effects on the human body are not identical to the estrogens produced by the ovaries, they offer the same benefits. They are used to manage hot flashes and the genitourinary effects of menopause and to reduce the risk of osteoporosis.

Not all HRT preparations include progesterone or progesterone-like substances (progestins), collectively called progestogens. However, if you would like to use HRT and have an intact uterus, it is advisable to include progestogens to support the health of your uterus. Apart from the benefits for the uterus, progesterone is also beneficial for managing the sleep disturbances and mood swings associated with menopause, and it may offer protection for breast tissue.

Both estrogen and progesterone can be taken orally in the form of a pill. Alternatively, they can be absorbed through the skin from transdermal patches. Although not approved by the FDA, there are also preparations such as progesterone creams and vaginal inserts available that may be useful during menopause. There is little to no scientific evidence to support the use of these products. Therefore, should you consider using them, it is advisable to get advice from your healthcare practitioner first.

Like all modern medicines, HRT comes with a list of pros and cons. While it can be a lifesaver for many women, the risks associated with using it are too high for others. Below is a list of pros and cons to help you decide if HRT is a good menopause management choice.

Pros:

1. **Symptom Relief:** HRT is highly effective in alleviating common menopausal symptoms, such as hot flashes, night sweats, and mood swings.

2. **Bone Health:** Estrogen helps maintain bone density, reducing the risk of osteoporosis.

3. **Vaginal Health:** HRT can address vaginal dryness and discomfort,

improving overall genitourinary health.

Cons:

1. **Health Risks:** Long-term use of HRT may be associated with increased risks of breast cancer, heart disease, and blood clots. The decision to use HRT should be personalized, considering an individual's medical history and risk factors.

2. **Individual Variability:** Responses to HRT vary among women, and not everyone experiences the same benefits. Regular monitoring is crucial to assess the ongoing appropriateness of the therapy.

Before considering HRT, women should have an in-depth discussion with their healthcare provider so they can make informed decisions based on their unique health profile (Harper-Harrison, n.d.).

Nutritional Supplements

A healthy, balanced diet goes a long way towards reducing the symptoms of menopause and minimizing the risk of chronic conditions such as heart disease and osteoporosis, as you will see in Chapter Seven. However, it is not always possible to meet your nutritional requirements through diet alone. As such, there are certain nutrients you may need to supplement to ensure you are consuming as much as your body needs to be healthy.

Useful nutritional supplements during menopause include:

Calcium

Calcium is essential for maintaining bone mineral density to prevent osteoporosis. The recommended daily calcium intake is 1,200 mg from food or a combination of food and supplements. Calcium can be found in dairy products, leafy greens, and almonds.

Vitamin D

Vitamin D is critical for calcium absorption, contributing to bone health. It is recommended that women obtain 400 - 600 IU of vitamin D from a combination of sun exposure, dietary sources, and supplements. Vitamin D can be found in oily fish like salmon, liver, egg yolks, and red meat.

Omega-3 Fatty Acids

Essential fatty acids, especially omega-3, may benefit women during menopause. They are anti-inflammatory and reduce the risk of chronic conditions like heart disease and diabetes. Moreover, omega-3 fatty acids have been shown to help menopausal women manage symptoms such as hot flashes, depression, and brain fog (Ciappolino et al., 2018). The exact dose of omega-3 for managing menopausal symptoms is unclear. Research suggests an intake of between 1,000 and 1,500 mg daily is needed (Dempsey et al., 2023). Omega-3 can be found in fatty fish (e.g., salmon, mackerel), flaxseeds, and walnuts.

Magnesium

Magnesium is involved in more than 300 chemical reactions throughout the body. While magnesium deficiency is rare in people eating a balanced diet, requirements may be increased during menopause. For example, studies have found that women with a higher magnesium intake are less likely to have depressive symptoms than those with a low magnesium intake. In addition, magnesium is important for bone health as it may help reduce bone loss. There is also a link between low magnesium levels and high blood pressure (Porri et al., 2021). The recommended daily intake is around 320 mg for women over 30 (*Magnesium - Health Professional Fact Sheet*, n.d.). Magnesium can be found in nuts, seeds, whole grains, and leafy green vegetables.

Vitamin E

Although not as effective as HRT, vitamin E supplementation has been shown to reduce hot flashes, improve cholesterol levels, and help manage the vaginal changes that occur during menopause (Feduniw et al., 2022). The recommended daily intake is around 15 mg. Vitamin E can be found in nuts, seeds, and vegetable oils.

Probiotics for Gut Health

In the last 20 – 30 years, the importance of gut health has been recognized for the benefits it offers for all parts of your body. Not only does a healthy digestive system ensure that your food is digested and nutrients absorbed, but it also impacts your metabolism, immunity, and brain health. While the proper structure and function of the cells, enzymes, and hormones of your digestive tract are critical for gut health, the colony of microorganisms, collectively known as the gut microbiome, also plays a significant role.

Did you know that you have more than 100 trillion microbes living within your gut? Even more amazing is that they are not simply hitching a free ride. Your gut bacteria have several important functions. First, they can digest dietary fiber, which the human digestive system cannot. In doing so, they release chemicals called short-chain fatty acids used as fuel by the cells lining the intestines. They also affect your metabolism, helping to control your blood sugar and cholesterol levels.

The more beneficial bacteria in your gut, the less chance there is of harmful bacteria growing out of control and causing digestive issues. Therefore, a balanced gut microbiome is essential for overall health (Valdes et al., 2018).

Although more research needs to be done, scientists have seen significant changes in the gut microbiome of menopausal women. As hormone levels drop, the diversity in the type of bacteria in the gut also declines, having a profound effect on women's gut health. Apart from factors like diet, immunity, disease, and antibiotic use, which are known to affect the gut microbiome, estrogen and progesterone also have a role to play in digestive health. The hormones help to protect the integrity of the gut lining, thus preventing the absorption of large molecules and microbes that usually do not enter the bloodstream.

However, it is not only the sex hormones that protect the gut. Certain types of bacteria can transform deactivated estrogen and progesterone that are destined for elimination into active forms of the hormones, which then reenter your bloodstream to be used again, thus helping to boost your hormone levels (Peters et al., 2022).

While a balanced fiber-rich diet and other lifestyle habits such as regular physical activity and getting enough sleep support a healthy gut, probiotic supplements may be useful to keep the balance in your gut microbiome in menopause. Lactic acid bacteria have shown promising results in scientific studies, suggesting that taking a supplement with these bacterial strains may help manage the signs and symptoms of menopause. Although more research is needed, probiotic supplements may help prevent bone loss, reduce vaginal symptoms, help regulate the nervous system, and improve the metabolism of fat, resulting in lower levels of fat in the blood (Chen et al., 2022).

Herbal Remedies

There are several natural remedies made from plants that may be useful in the management of menopause symptoms. Since they are prepared from roots, stems, leaves, or flowers instead of chemicals, they are considered food by the FDA. Therefore, they do not undergo the same rigorous testing as scientifically formulated medications such as HRT, and the manufacturing and labelling of such products are largely unregulated. Also, remember that all women are different, and an herbal preparation that works well for your friend may not offer the same benefits for you. For these reasons, it is recommended that you consult with a healthcare practitioner before taking an herbal supplement for your menopause symptoms to ensure that it is safe for you to use and won't interfere with any medication you are taking.

When choosing an herbal supplement, consider the brand's reputation and whether the product has been independently tested. Third-party testing is a way of confirming that the product contains all the ingredients listed on the label in the amounts specified. Also, look for supplements using standardized extracts to ensure dosage consistency. Different methods of preparation and varieties in the plants contribute to varying levels of the active ingredients in a natural product (*Herbal Medicine | Johns Hopkins Medicine*, 2021).

The herbal remedies listed below may help ease your midlife transition. While they have all been included in scientific studies on the possible benefits of herbal supplements for managing menopausal symptoms, there is insufficient research to say without a doubt that they are safe and effective. Some studies conclude that such supplements are safe and effective, and yet others find no benefits (Johnson et al., 2019).

Black Cohosh

Used as a traditional medicine for the management of hot flashes, mood swings, and other menopausal symptoms, Black Cohosh is a popular herbal remedy that has been widely studied. Supplements are made from the roots of the *Cimicifuga racemose* plant and are available in many forms, including powdered and liquid extracts. However, there is little evidence to prove that it is effective, especially when taken on its own. It may be beneficial when combined with other herbs like St John's Wort (*Black Cohosh - Health Professional Fact Sheet*, n.d.). The recommended intake varies between 20-40 mg daily, but individual responses vary. Black Cohosh is safe for most women to use. It may cause temporary side effects like gastrointestinal upsets such as nausea, diarrhea, and skin rashes.

Dong Quai

The ancient Chinese herb Dong Quai is made from the roots of the Angelica sinensis plant. It is available in pills, capsules, powders, and liquid preparations and is known for potentially relieving menstrual symptoms and menopausal discomfort. However, studies examining the herb's effects on menopausal symptoms offer conflicting results. When used on its own, Dong Quai does not seem to offer any benefits for menopausal women. Even so, there is some evidence to suggest that using it in conjunction with other herbs, such as Black Cohosh, may increase its effectiveness (Johnson et al., 2019). There are no standardized guidelines for the amount of Dong Quai you should take. General recommendations suggest three to six grams per day. While considered safe, Dong Quai may interact with other herbs and medication. Other side effects include sun sensitivity and blood clotting issues.

Maca

Maca is a cruciferous root vegetable used as a food and medicine for boosting energy levels, balancing hormones, managing menopause symptoms, and improving thyroid function in native Peruvian cultures. Scientists think the effects of this plant therapy are a result of chemicals called plant sterols acting on the endocrine system rather than hormones present in the maca. Although more studies need to be done to confirm the benefits and safety profile of this menopausal remedy, initial research has yielded promising results (Brooks et al., 2008). Research suggests women take two grams of Maca daily to alleviate menopause symptoms. Maca is generally safe to use for most women but should be avoided during pregnancy and breastfeeding. Most side effects are temporary and include indigestion, bloating, and gas. Talk to your healthcare provider before taking maca if you have any hormone-sensitive conditions such as breast cancer, endometriosis, and ovarian cancer (*Maca: MedlinePlus Supplements*, n.d.).

Red Clover

The phytoestrogens, or plant forms of estrogen, found in red clover may help reduce menopausal symptoms such as hot flashes. However, research shows mixed results (Johnson et al., 2019). 40 mg of red clover was given to women in a study that showed reduced hot flashes because of the natural remedy and can be used as a daily recommended intake limit. Red clover is safe to use for 12 months. Side effects may include skin rashes, nausea, and headaches.

Wild Yam

Used in Traditional Chinese Medicine for treating menopausal symptoms, wild yam may be useful for relief from hot flashes and mood disorders associated with dropping hormone levels. Even so, there are very few scientific studies on natural therapy and its possible benefits for women during menopause. The results of the research that has been done have been mixed (Johnson et al., 2019). Research suggests that 12mg of wild yam may offer relief from the symptoms of menopause.Wild yam is typically well tolerated for up to 12 weeks. Side effects may include headaches and an upset stomach. Women with hormone-sensitive conditions such as breast cancer, endometriosis, and ovarian cancer must consult with their healthcare practitioner before using wild yam.

It is crucial to note that while natural remedies can offer relief, their effectiveness varies among individuals. Therefore, you must consult your healthcare professional before incorporating these supplements into your menopause management plan.

In conclusion, managing menopause demands a personalized approach to treat your unique set of symptoms and health issues in midlife. Whether you are considering hormone replacement therapy, nutritional supplements, natural remedies, or a combination of therapies, collaborating with your healthcare provider can help you find the best management options. Being aware of your choices ensures that you can make informed decisions that promote your health and well-being during this transformative phase of life.

SELF-ASSESSMENT AND TESTING FOR MENOPAUSE

The way women experience menopause varies. Even though the onset of symptoms is typically gradual, beginning with subtle changes, as your hormone levels continue to drop, they become more noticeable and debilitating. In the spirit of being "forearmed is forewarned", knowing what to look out for can help you develop a management plan before your symptoms become overwhelming.

For this reason, Chapter Six offers guidance on assessing your menopause status, from being mindful of your menstrual cycle to paying attention to your mood, energy levels, and changes to your skin and hair. Blood tests for assessing your levels of estrogen and progesterone will also be discussed, along with thyroid function tests and bone density scans.

Simple Self-Assessments to Understand Hormonal Status

Self-awareness is key to assessing your hormonal status. It involves being mindful of several aspects of your health. That said, it must be noted that although the self-assessment guide below is a useful tool for understanding your health in midlife, it is not a substitute for professional medical advice. It is essential to consult with your doctor if your symptoms are affecting your quality of life or if you have any specific health concerns.

Answer the questions in this self-assessment tool based on the information you have learned up to this point to gain clarity on your menstrual cycle, hormone-related symptoms, lifestyle habits, sexual health, and overall health and well-being.

Menstrual Health

Menstrual Cycle Regularity:

Are your menstrual cycles regular, occurring roughly every 21 to 35 days? Do you experience any irregularities, such as missed periods or frequent spotting?

Menstrual Flow:

Is your menstrual flow light, moderate, or heavy? Have you noticed any significant changes in flow over the last few months?

Pain and Discomfort:

Rate the severity of any menstrual cramps or discomfort on a scale of 1 to 10. Are there specific times during your cycle when you experience increased pain?

Explanation: As you already know, your ovaries handle making and releasing estrogen, and the number of follicles in your ovaries drops with each menstrual cycle. As a result of fluctuating estrogen levels during perimenopause, you may experience some changes in your menstrual cycle. The further you get along the path to menopause, the more obvious the changes become. Initially, your menstrual cycle may be a few days longer or shorter than it was before, and the flow may be heavier or lighter. Eventually, you will begin skipping periods. Once you have gone a full year with no menstrual bleeding, you are in menopause.

Hormonal Symptoms

Mood and Emotions:

Have you noticed any mood changes, like having a low mood or feeling more anxious than normal?
Does it feel like you have no control over your emotions?

Energy Levels:

Describe your energy levels throughout the month. Have you noticed any changes in your energy levels?

Skin and Hair Changes:

Have you observed any changes in your skin, like acne, dryness, or itching? Are you experiencing hair loss or dry, brittle hair?

Changing hormone levels can leave you feeling low and anxious. You may also experience what many women refer to as "meno-rage", when you feel like you have no control over your anger and snap at anyone and everyone. Whether you lose your temper more regularly or cry while watching endearing commercials, your emotions seem to develop a mind of their own during perimenopause. Add to that a general feeling of fatigue, dry skin, and thinning hair, it is no wonder people think middle aged women are a little crazy.

Lifestyle Factors

Exercise Routine:

Do you include physical activity in your daily routine? Has your exercise capacity changed? For example, has your muscle strength dropped, or can you run at the same pace as you did before?

Diet and Nutrition:

Keep a food diary for a week. Include everything you eat, how you feel when you eat, how you feel after meals, and why you eat. Also, record any food cravings and everything you drink. Has your appetite changed? Are you eating the same amount, more, or less than before?

Sleep Patterns:

Describe your sleep patterns and quality. Do you find it easy to fall asleep? Do you wake up during the night or too early in the morning?

Healthy lifestyle habits can help you manage your menopausal symptoms. Making time for regular physical activity, eating a healthy diet, and getting enough good quality sleep can help boost your mood and support your overall health. However, declining hormone levels can make it harder to motivate yourself to lace up your sneakers and get some exercise due to increased fatigue. Hormones also affect your appetite. During perimenopause, many women have increased cravings for sweet foods and eat more than they need to, contributing to weight gain. Furthermore, your hormone levels may start affecting your sleeping habits. It might become more difficult to fall asleep, or you may find yourself lying awake at 2 am, unable to go back to sleep.

Sexual Health

Vaginal Health:

Have you noticed any changes to your vagina, such as dryness or itching? Has sexual intercourse become painful? Are you experiencing more vaginal or urinary tract infections?

Libido:

Has your desire to be intimate with your partner changed?

As you know, a drop in estrogen and progesterone profoundly affects your genitourinary system. It may result in thinning of the vaginal wall and reduced production of moisture, causing dryness and itching. Consequently, sex may become painful, and the risk of vaginal and urinary tract infections increases during menopause. Furthermore, declining levels of sex hormones cause a drop in your libido, reducing your desire to be intimate with your partner.

General Health and Wellness

Overall Well-being:

Rate your overall well-being on a scale of one to ten. Are there specific concerns or symptoms affecting your daily life?

The list of possible symptoms caused by a drop in estrogen and progesterone is extensive. While not all changes in your body will result from changing hormone levels, many of them could be. Consult with your healthcare provider if you are experiencing worrying changes in your overall health and well-being.

Assessing your health and probable hormone status is a useful place to start. However, it may be necessary to do some blood work to establish exactly where you stand. When you talk to your doctor, describe all your symptoms, even if you think they are irrelevant, and share your concerns about your health and menopause. They will then be able to help you with the appropriate blood tests that will give you insight into which stage of menopause you are in and whether you are at risk of developing any chronic conditions such as diabetes or osteoporosis.

Recommended Lab Testing

An annual health check helps ensure that any health problems are caught early, enabling you to treat them before they become a serious problem. Several preventive screening tools are recommended for women between 40 and 64. For instance, women should have regular mammograms every one to two years to screen for breast cancer and a pap smear every three years to check for cervical cancer. Your doctor will check your blood pressure at every consultation, and depending on your risk factors, they may request a battery of blood tests to investigate signs of high cholesterol and raised blood sugar levels (*Health Screenings for Women Ages 40 to 64: MedlinePlus Medical Encyclopedia*, n.d.).

To assess your menopausal status, your doctor may request the following blood tests:

Hormone panels

A hormone panel is a set of blood tests that measures the levels of various hormones in a woman's blood. These tests are commonly used to assess hormonal status and identify any imbalances that may contribute to health issues or symptoms of menopause. The specific hormones included in a hormone panel can vary, but hormone panels typically include the following tests:

Estradiol: Checking estradiol levels helps evaluate your menstrual cycle, fertility, and menopausal status. Normal levels of this hormone vary depending on your life stage. During adolescence, levels range between 20 – 300 pg/ml (picograms per milliliter); when you are pregnant, estradiol levels can be over 20,000 pg/ml, and after menopause, levels drop significantly to less than 20 pg/ml (Stanczyk & Clarke, 2014).

Progesterone: Since progesterone levels change significantly between the beginning of your menstrual cycle and the days following ovulation, blood tests are used to evaluate the second half of your menstrual cycle and to assess fertility and pregnancy. It is generally not useful for predicting your menopausal status. However, after menopause, progesterone levels are very low – less than 0.2 nanograms per milliliter (Cable, n.d.).

Follicle-Stimulating Hormone (FSH): Levels of this hormone vary depending on where you are in your menstrual cycle. FSH levels are measured in milli-international units per milliliter (mIU/ml). At the beginning of your cycle FSH levels should be between 1.4 – 9.9 mIU/ml, during ovulation they can be between 6.2 – 17.2 mIU/ml, and before your period, they may drop to 1.1 – 9.2 mIU/ml. Elevated levels of 19.3 – 100.6 mIU/ml may indicate menopause or ovarian dysfunction (*Follicle-Stimulating Hormone - Health Encyclopedia - University of Rochester Medical Center*, n.d.).

Luteinizing Hormone (LH): Levels of luteinizing hormone fluctuate with your menstrual cycle. At the beginning of your cycle, LH levels typically fall between 1.68 – 15 IU/ml (International units per milliliter), mid-cycle it rises to between 21.9 – 56.6 IU/ml, and before your period, it drops to 0.61 – 16.3 IU/ml. After menopause, luteinizing hormone levels range between 14.2 – 52.3 IU/ml

(*Luteinizing Hormone (Blood) - Health Encyclopedia - University of Rochester Medical Center*, n.d.).

Thyroid Stimulating Hormone (TSH): Blood levels of TSH are used to evaluate thyroid function. The normal range for TSH is 0.5 – 5.0 mIU/ml. Raised levels of this hormone are a sign of an underactive thyroid gland (hypothyroidism). This result is used in combination with your free T4 and free T3 results to determine how well your thyroid gland is working (*Normal Thyroid Hormone Levels - Endocrine Surgery | UCLA Health*, n.d.).

Free T4 (Thyroxine): Thyroxine measures the level of active thyroid hormone in the blood. The normal range is 5 – 12 micrograms per deciliter (mg/dl)

Free T3 (Triiodothyronine): The test measures the active form of Free T3, the thyroid hormone, in your blood. The normal range is 80 – 220 ng/dl.

Testosterone and Sex Hormone-Binding Globulin (SHBG): Testosterone levels in women are difficult to measure accurately as most of the testosterone is bound to sex hormone-binding globulin. Therefore, the laboratory may use an equation that involves the values of free testosterone and sex hormone-binding globulin to calculate whether your testosterone levels are low (Scott & Newson, 2020).

When considered together, these hormone tests provide valuable information about your reproductive health, thyroid function, and overall hormonal balance. However, the interpretation of hormone levels is complex and must be considered with your specific symptoms and medical history. A healthcare provider, often an endocrinologist or gynecologist, can help interpret these results and suggest appropriate interventions.

Bone density scans

Bone density scans, also known as dual-energy X-ray absorptiometry scans (DEXA or DXA), are medical tests used to measure the density of your bones to assess bone strength and risk of fractures.

Purpose of Bone Density Scans:

1. **Diagnosing osteoporosis:** Bone density scans are commonly used to diagnose osteoporosis and assess the severity of the condition. The results help doctors determine the risk of fractures and guide treatment decisions (*Bone Density Scan: MedlinePlus Medical Test*, n.d.).

2. **Determine your risk of bone fractures:** By measuring bone density, these scans provide information about the risk of fractures in different body areas. This information is crucial for developing preventive strate-

gies and managing overall bone health.

3. **Monitoring bone health:** Bone density scans can be used to monitor changes in bone density over time. This is particularly important for individuals undergoing treatment for osteoporosis or other conditions affecting bone health.

When and How Often to Get Tested

Your age, symptoms, and medical history will determine when and how often your doctor will suggest testing your hormone levels and screening for other conditions, including breast and cervical cancer, high blood pressure, heart disease, diabetes, and osteoporosis. In some cases, such tests may be part of your routine preventive care, while in others, they may be suggested based on specific health concerns. Developing a relationship with your healthcare provider is crucial for effectively managing menopausal symptoms. When you feel comfortable discussing your health with your doctor, and they understand you and your personal health concerns, you can work together to manage your symptoms in midlife and prevent chronic diseases.

THE IMPORTANCE OF NUTRITION DURING MENOPAUSE

G ood nutrition is the foundation of human health. As such, your body thrives when you eat the right nutrients in the right amounts. With that in mind, you may be wondering if your nutritional requirements change during the menopause transition. After all, your waistline seems to be increasing uncontrollably, and your doctor may have told you your blood pressure and glucose levels are climbing.

Since estrogen and progesterone have a significant impact on many systems and functions throughout your body, your question is one hundred percent valid. Not only do you experience metabolic changes when your hormone levels start declining, resulting in the dreaded middle-age spread, but you may also have to manage new health issues as a result.

Although diet can't address or help manage all the physiological effects of menopause, it can help you manage your weight, improve your flagging energy levels, and control your blood sugar and insulin levels. Since lower estrogen levels can also cause increased levels of inflammation in your body, eating foods that reduce chronic inflammation is a useful tactic for reducing the impact of the transition on your overall health and well-being.

In general, many women have a love-hate relationship with food and turn to dieting when the weight gain that seems inevitable during perimenopause creeps up on them. Unfortunately, extreme calorie restriction or cutting out entire food groups to lose weight may do more harm than good. Your body is less resilient in your late forties and early fifties than it was in your younger years, and your changing hormones make it more challenging to deal with the physical and emotional stress of dieting.

Menopause is hard enough without punishing yourself with a strict diet. So, let's explore the nutrients your body needs during menopause and how to create a more mindful meal plan that meets your body's needs while preventing weight gain and managing new health conditions.

Nutritional Requirements During Menopause

Your basic dietary requirements during menopause are similar to what they have been up to this point. Even though your body is changing, it still requires a balance of essential nutrients and energy to maintain the structure and function of all organs and systems. Therefore, your diet should be based on the following dietary guidelines (*Dietary Guidelines for Americans, 2020-2025 and Online Materials | Dietary Guidelines for Americans*, n.d.):

- Eat a variety of colorful vegetables, preferably with every meal. Aim for three to five cups per day.

- Include fruit in your meal plan every day. You can enjoy two to three fruits per day.

- Eat whole-grain carbohydrates such as brown rice, barley, and oats with most meals.

- Consume two to three portions of dairy products such as yogurt, cheese, and milk daily.

- Ensure every meal contains a source of protein, whether it is animal-based, such as meat, fish, chicken, and eggs, or plant-based, including beans, lentils, and chickpeas.

- Fats and oils contribute essential fatty acids to your diet. Include moderate amounts of omega-3-rich oils such as canola, olive, and avocado oil.

One of the easiest ways to bring these guidelines together is the food plate model (*USDA MyPlate What Is MyPlate?*, n.d.). Instead of weighing and measuring everything you eat, which no one has time for, divide your plate into quarters. Fill half your plate with vegetables, a quarter with carbohydrate foods, and the remaining quarter with protein. That is approximately equal to two fists of veggies, one fist of carbs, and a palm-sized portion of protein.

The fat portion of your meals will most likely be used during the cooking process, but you can, of course, drizzle some olive oil or toasted sunflower seeds over your salad, for example, if you are missing the fat factor.

For fruit, you can enjoy it as part of your meals or as a snack between meals, and the same is true for dairy products. It is a common misconception that fruit contains too much sugar and is, therefore, bad for weight loss. Luckily, that's not true. There is no need to worry about the sugar in fruit as it comes packaged with dietary fiber to slow down the release of sugar into the blood and nutrients to support your overall health.

Eating for Bone Health

Osteoporosis is no laughing matter. Unfortunately, although estrogen has a protective effect on bone mineral density, when levels start to decline, the loss of bone density increases the risk of fractures. That makes calcium, vitamin D, magnesium, vitamin K, and protein essential for menopausal women.

Calcium

Calcium forms the bulk of the structure of our bones. In addition, the calcium in the bones is released to maintain the levels of minerals in the blood, which are used to support nerve structure and healthy muscle contractions. Our calcium requirements differ from one life stage to the next, depending on growth. Since the rate at which calcium is lost from the bones increases when women enter menopause, their calcium requirements are greater than men's after the age of 50. It is recommended that menopausal women consume 1,200mg of calcium per day (*Calcium Content of Common Foods | International Osteoporosis Foundation*, n.d.).

Sources of calcium include the following:

- Dairy products (milk, cheese, and yogurt)
- Green leafy vegetables (broccoli, spinach, and kale)
- Fruits (oranges, papaya, and apricots)
- Nuts (almonds and hazelnuts)
- Seeds (sesame seeds)
- Seafood (canned sardines with bones, shrimp, and canned tuna with bones)
- Legumes (white beans, chickpeas, and lentils)
- Soya products (tofu)

Vitamin D

Our primary source of vitamin D is the sun. Exposing your skin to the sun's UV rays triggers the synthesis of vitamin D in your body in the form of vitamin D3, also called cholecalciferol. To make enough vitamin D to meet your body's needs and promote the absorption of calcium to build strong bones, you must expose the bare skin of your face, arms, and hands to the sun, preferably before 10 am and after 2 pm, every day. Remember that to benefit from the sun's rays, they need access to your skin. That means no clothing or sunscreen. Therefore, avoiding the midday sun is recommended to avoid sunburn.

Unfortunately, we can't always count on the sun for this essential vitamin. If you live in an environment that receives very little sunshine, for example, or you have sensitive skin, you will have to find your vitamin D elsewhere. It seems obvious that you should turn to food. After all, your food is the source of other essential nutrients, but there are very few food sources of vitamin D. You may find milk that is fortified with the sunshine vitamin, but not all milk will contain significant levels (*Vitamin D | International Osteoporosis Foundation*, n.d.):

There are some foods you can include in your diet to boost your vitamin D levels. They include:

- Sun-dried shitake mushrooms (When you leave mushrooms in the sun, they produce more vitamin D, like humans. So, whenever you cook with mushrooms, not only shitake mushrooms, chop them up and set them out to sunbathe for 15 minutes to 2 hours before cooking them (Cardwell et al., 2018)

- Wild-caught salmon

- Canned sardines

Magnesium

Magnesium is an essential mineral in the human diet and involves over 300 chemical pathways in the body. It is an important component in maintaining bone strength. As such, adequate amounts of magnesium must be included in your diet (Rondanelli et al., 2021).

Good sources of magnesium include:

- Green leafy vegetables (broccoli, spinach, and kale)
- Legumes (beans, chickpeas, and lentils)
- Nuts (Brazil nuts, cashews, and almonds)
- Seeds (chia, pumpkin, and sunflower)
- Whole grains (wheat, barley, and oats)

Vitamin K

Although vitamin K is well-known for its role in blood coagulation, it is an essential nutrient for maintaining healthy bones. It can be found in dark green leafy vegetables such as spinach and kale, dairy products, egg yolk, and liver (Elshaikh et al., 2020).

Eating for Heart Health

Estrogen has a protective effect on a woman's cardiovascular system. Consequently, as estrogen levels start to drop, it is common for women to develop high cholesterol levels and high blood pressure (hypertension).

Although the primary cause of these conditions during midlife is changes in hormone levels, diet plays a role in managing them. As such, eating a heart-healthy diet is highly recommended for women in the menopausal transition and post-menopause (Ryczkowska et al., 2022).

The following heart-healthy dietary guidelines are recommended by the American Heart Association(*The American Heart Association Diet and Lifestyle Recommendations*, 2021):

- Eat the rainbow. In other words, include a wide variety of fruits and vegetables of different colors in your diet every day.

- Replace refined carbohydrates with whole-grain foods.

- Choose lean protein sources such as lean red meat, skinless chicken, fish, and plant-based proteins such as beans, lentils, and chickpeas.

- Limit the amount of fat you add to your food, especially saturated fat. Instead, choose oils such as olive, canola, and avocado oil.

- Eat more whole foods than processed foods. Ultra-processed foods, such as deli meats, sugary breakfast cereals, mass-produced bread, and instant soups, generally have a higher fat, sugar, and salt content than minimally processed foods, such as lean cold meat, oatmeal, sourdough bread, and homemade soup.

- Limit your intake of added sugars by eating chocolate, sweets, and baked goods as occasional treats and opting for water instead of sugar-filled soft drinks.

- Reduce the amount of salt you add to food. As a general rule, either cook with salt or add it later at the table. Remember that foods such as potato chips, soup powders, pre-cooked meals, and canned foods have a high salt content.

- Drink alcohol only in moderation.

Phyto Estrogens

Several plant compounds have a similar structure to estrogen, referred to as phyto (plant) estrogens. When you eat them, they are metabolized by the bacteria in the gut, absorbed into the bloodstream, and processed in the liver. They have a similar effect on the body as the estrogen your body produces. As such, they have been investigated as a way to help women manage menopause. One of the most effective phyto estrogens is isoflavones, commonly found in legumes, with soybeans having the highest concentration. Therefore, adding soya products to your diet can help you manage menopause symptoms. As such, tofu, soya milk, and edamame beans can be a useful addition to your diet.

Food sources of other phyto estrogens include peanuts, grapes, garlic, carrots, potatoes, whole wheat, apples, and coffee. The concentration of plant estrogens in such foods is low, so they are less beneficial than the isoflavones found in soy (Desmawati & Sulastri, 2019).

Note about breast cancer and soy isoflavones:

Many women are hesitant to include soy in their diet due to the belief that it may contribute to the development of breast cancer. While high levels of estrogen trigger some types of breast cancer, the level of phytoestrogens in soy is too low for it to be a problem. A scientific study that examined the results of 8 research papers on the topic of soy isoflavones and breast cancer found that rather than causing breast cancer, consuming soy products may protect both pre- and post-menopausal women from the disease (BOUTAS et al., 2022). However, while soy is considered safe and is an excellent source of protein and dietary fiber, you do not have to include it your diet if you are concerned about the possibility of it contributing to your risk of breast cancer.

Caffeine and Alcohol

Think back to the last cup of coffee you drank. It was just what the doctor ordered. It gave you the lift you were craving. But... was it followed by the rising heat of a hot flush that had you removing your jersey, tying back your hair, and fanning yourself with the nearest thing you could find to move the air around? While the moderate intake of caffeine is not harmful, even the smallest amount can trigger those unpleasant vasomotor symptoms the majority of women experience during perimenopause and menopause. If hot flushes are a significant problem for you, it may be better, or at least more comfortable, for you to limit your caffeine intake (Faubion et al., 2015).

What about your evening glass of wine? Do you have to go without? Life is miserable enough with all the menopause symptoms you must contend with every day. Surely, you can still enjoy your sundowner. The simple answer is, yes, you can still enjoy a glass of wine at the end of the day. However, it should only be one glass, and a small one at that – just five fluid ounces (150ml). If you are a beer drinker, that is the equivalent of one bottle or can, and if you drink spirits, it's just a single shot. According to The North American Menopause Society, moderate drinking, as described above, can be beneficial for women. It may reduce your risk of heart disease, diabetes, and dementia and improve your bone strength.

However, when you drink more than one drink per day, your drinking habit may increase your risk of breast cancer and heart disease and result in weight gain, especially around your middle. In addition, it can trigger hot flashes and worsen symptoms of depression (*Alcohol & Menopause, Menopause Information & Articles | The North American Menopause Society, NAMS*, n.d.).

The Importance of Nutrition During Menopause

In your twenties and thirties, your body was more adaptable. You could eat and drink almost whatever you wanted, and if you gained a bit of weight, it was easier to lose. Now that you're in your forties or fifties, things have changed. It seems that just walking past a bakery will make you gain five pounds, and recovering after a night out drinking takes a lot longer. Estrogen was your best friend. It is used to help you metabolize your meals more effectively, and it protects you from chronic diseases. As the levels of this amazing female hormone drop, your metabolism slows down, and your selection of the food and drink you choose to consume must be more deliberate.

Eating a healthy, balanced diet not only helps you maintain your weight and reduces your risk of developing chronic health conditions, but it also improves your menopause symptoms.

Weight Management Strategies in Midlife

B ecause menopause is a gradual shift in hormone levels, you may not notice your weight climbing at first. Nevertheless, slowly but surely, your clothes start fitting a bit more snuggly, and you start feeling the extra fat on your belly when you sit down. Then, suddenly, it seems that every time you step on the scale, the number gets higher and higher.

Considering all the other less-than-delightful side effects of menopause, it's not fair that you now must watch what you eat more closely to avoid middle-age spread. To add to the problem, it can feel like no matter what you eat and how careful you are, nothing makes a difference.

Don't give up in despair. Weight loss may be more challenging during menopause, but it is not impossible. While you may never again be the weight you were in your early twenties, you don't have to resign yourself to becoming obese.

Importance of Maintaining a Healthy Weight

Maintaining a healthy weight is important at any life stage. However, as you get older and your hormones start playing games with you and your health, striving to be in good shape becomes crucial.

As we discussed in Chapter Four, declining levels of estrogen increase your risk of chronic health conditions such as cardiovascular disease and type 2 diabetes. Unfortunately, it also results in weight gain, which is associated with similar health risks.

The Centers for Disease Control and Prevention (CDC) reports that people with a BMI over 25 are at greater risk of dying from any cause. They are also more likely to have high blood pressure, raised cholesterol levels, type 2 diabetes, joint problems, sleep apnea, osteoarthritis, and gallbladder disease (*Health Effects of Overweight and Obesity | Healthy Weight, Nutrition, and Physical Activity | CDC*, 2022).

Generally, the body mass index (BMI) determines whether your weight is ideal, too low, or too high. It may not be the best tool as it is based on your height and weight and doesn't consider how much lean muscle and body fat you have. However, it gives you an idea of whether your body weight is within the healthy range or not (*About Adult BMI | Healthy Weight, Nutrition, and Physical Activity | CDC*, 2022).

Here's the breakdown of BMI categories:

- Underweight: <18.5
- Healthy weight: 18.5 - 24.9
- Overweight: 25 - 29.9
- Obese: >30

Use the following calculations to work out your BMI:

Metric:

BMI = weight (kg) / height (m)^2
For example, If you are 175cm (1.75m) tall and weigh 68kg.
$BMI = 68 / (1.75 \times 1.75)$
$= 68 / 3.06$
$= 22.2 \, kg/m^2$

Pounds and inches:

BMI = weight (lb.) / height (in)^2 x 703
For example, if you are 5'6" and weigh 180 pounds,
$BMI = (180 / (66 \times 66)) \times 703$
$= (180 / 4356) \times 703$
$= 0.41 \times 703 = 29$

However, being overweight is not a cause for panic. You do not have to start starving yourself because you have gained a few pounds in midlife. Instead, stick to a healthy, balanced diet that meets your body's nutritional and energy requirements. At the very least, you can prevent further weight gain, and hopefully, you can shift the extra weight with time.

How to Choose the Right Diet

There is no such thing as the perfect diet that works for everyone. Your dietary requirements are as unique to you as your fingerprints. The best diet is one you can stick with for the long haul, developing healthy habits that will last you a lifetime. That said, there are several basic principles common to all healthy eating plans, whether they are low-carbohydrate, high-fat, high-protein, or vegan. Research suggests that a primarily plant-based diet consisting of various fruits and vegetables and whole grains served alongside either animal- or plant-based protein promotes good health (Katz & Meller, 2014). Even so, some women find it easiest to lose weight when restricting their carbohydrate intake, while others fare better on a low-fat diet. For many, a general calorie restriction works best, but others find an intermittent fasting routine works best.

To choose the right diet for you, you must ask yourself the following questions:

- Does the meal plan fit into your budget?

- Do you have enough time to prepare the meals?

- Do you have the cooking skills required to implement the meal plan?

- Does the type of food included in the diet suit your personal food preferences and your family's?

- Can your family follow the same diet?

- How much weight do you need to lose?

- Is the diet balanced, and will it support your health in midlife?

- What type of diet has worked best for you in the past?

- Is the diet flexible? Will you be able to follow the diet even when you are pressed for time, at a conference, or on a family vacation?

- Is the diet very restrictive? In other words, will following it make you feel deprived and increase your food cravings?

Meal Planning and Preparation Tips

Whether your preferred diet is vegan, low-fat, or a more conventional plan that includes a variety of foods from all the food groups, sticking to it is easier if you have a plan and some simple preparation tricks up your sleeve. Given that most women have several balls to juggle the middle years of their lives, your diet shouldn't make things even more complicated.

The first step is to have a plan. You could consult with a registered dietitian or nutritionist to draw up an eating plan for you, or you could use one of the many dieting and fitness apps to guide you. Alternatively, if you feel confident about your dietary requirements, you could spend a little time creating a meal plan for yourself based on the general dietary guidelines. Whichever path you choose, having a plan sets you up for success.

The next step is to spend half an hour every week creating your menu. For those busy with work and family responsibilities or dread the time they have to spend in the kitchen, a basic rotation of meals works well. Try to include a range of proteins and vary your carbohydrates and vegetables throughout the week. For the more adventurous cooks who thrive on trying new recipes, you can plan a different meal for every day of the month.

Step three is to create a shopping list from your menu. Remember to take it with you when you go shopping! (Menopause brain fog is real.) Buy everything you need for the next few days or the whole week so when you get home after a long day, you have all the ingredients to whip up a healthy meal simply.

Meal prep ideas:

Let's face it: life is busy enough without spending hours in the kitchen every day. To solve that problem, meal preparation has become very popular. All the cool kids on social media are doing it... and so are the midlife moms!

It doesn't have to be a big commitment. You can prepare as much of your food in advance as you have the energy for, be it a few chopped veggies you can take out of the fridge at dinner time, or two to three complete meals to keep in your freezer for busy weekdays.

The following is a list of items that make meal prep a breeze:

- Ziplock bags
- Clean glass jars with tight-fitting lids
- Reusable plastic pouches
- Microwave and freezer-proof glass containers with tight-fitting lids
- Plastic food storage containers

Having the necessary equipment is one thing, but keeping your pantry stocked with cooking basics goes a long way to alleviating cooking-related stress. Always keep the following basics in your pantry:

- Salt
- Pepper

- A choice of herbs and spices
- Spaghetti and macaroni, or pasta of your choice
- Brown rice, wholewheat couscous, and barley
- All-purpose and corn flour
- Chicken, vegetable, and beef stock
- Olive oil
- Vinegar
- Canned tomatoes, tuna, beans, and chickpeas
- A selection of condiments and sauces
- Eggs
- Butter
- Milk
- Cheese
- Lemons
- Garlic
- Onions
- Potatoes
- Salad ingredients
- Meat, fish, and chicken (stored in the freezer)
- Frozen vegetables

Finally, here are some preparation ideas you can do every week to save you time:

- Prepare fresh vegetables for the week. Clean, peel, and chop them, then store them in airtight containers in the fridge.

- Prepare protein ingredients in advance for the week. Cut meat and chicken into the sizes needed for each meal and add marinade if it is part of the recipe. Place the prepared meat in Ziplock bags and store it in the fridge for two to three days or in the freezer for up to three months.

- Cook rice and other grains in bulk. Place as much as you need for a meal in individual freezer-proof containers and freeze them until needed.

- Cook for the fridge or freezer. It can save you a lot of time if you cook dishes like soups and stews in bulk and store them in the fridge or freezer until you need them. If you do this every time you cook a dish that freezes well, you will build up a stock of homemade convenience meals.

Your meal plan is your golden ticket to improved health and weight management during menopause. When you combine it with quick and easy meal preparation techniques, you become unstoppable.

One final note... don't punish yourself if your meal plan gets forgotten occasionally. No one can expect their diet to be perfect. There are days, sometimes many consecutive days, when you have to do whatever it takes to get through the day.

If that means eating the same simple meal several days in a row, then so be it. Tomorrow is another day.

DIETARY APPROACHES FOR MENOPAUSE

I t can be tempting when you're dealing with hot flushes and fatigue all day long, not to mention violent mood swings, to resort to quick, easy, convenience meals. After all, who has the energy to cook a healthy meal? However, the food you choose to eat makes a difference to how you experience the menopausal transition. When your body is well-nourished, the irritating and sometimes debilitating symptoms of "the change" can be mitigated.

The best diet for menopause is an individualized approach that seamlessly fits into your daily routine and nourishes your body and your brain. The eight diets summarized in this chapter are based on the basic nutrition guidelines, yet each one focuses on different aspects of diet and nutrition, offering unique benefits.

Whether you're in the middle of perimenopause or just starting to anticipate its arrival, understanding the role of your eating habits in managing your symptoms and promoting overall health is a crucial step in taking control of your well-being. If you feel a standard balanced diet is best for you, that's great. If you need to focus on chronic inflammation or heart health, you may want to consider a Mediterranean style of eating, the DASH diet, or an anti-inflammatory diet. Otherwise, if your focus is more on weight loss and blood sugar control, a low glycemic index diet or the ketogenic diet may be the most suitable choice for you.

You may need to adopt aspects of a combination of dietary approaches to find an eating plan that works for you and be flexible to allow it to develop over time. At the same time, your food is your friend. There is no need to feel guilty about having a chocolate binge or occasionally skipping your veggies. One less than ideal meal will not cause lasting damage.

Let's explore the scientifically backed dietary approaches to menopause that have proven benefits for weight management and general health and wellbeing.

#1 Balanced Diet

Everyone talks about eating a healthy, balanced diet, but what does that mean? In essence, a balanced diet is a way of eating that provides your body with all the energy and nutrients it needs to promote health. It includes eating a variety of foods from all the food groups: carbohydrates, fats, proteins, dairy products, and fruit and vegetables in the right amounts (Cena & Calder, 2020).

A balanced diet typically includes the following key components:

1. **Carbohydrates:** Carbohydrates are your body's main source of energy. All carbohydrates are broken down into sugar when they are digested, supplying energy in the form of glucose. In a balanced diet, 50-60% of your total daily calories can be in the form of carbohydrates. The best types of carbohydrate foods are high in fiber such as brown rice, whole wheat pasta, whole grain bread, rolled oats, and barley. Fiber is critical for gut health and managing blood sugar levels.

2. **Proteins:** Protein is an essential macronutrient and should make up 20% of your total daily calorie intake. It is responsible for building and repairing tissues such as muscle in the body, and it is a component of hormones, enzymes, and antibodies. Good sources of protein include lean meats, poultry, fish, beans, lentils, chickpeas, tofu, nuts, and dairy products.

3. **Fats:** Fat provides the body with twice as much energy per gram as carbohydrates. Therefore, only a small amount of fat is included in a balanced diet, approximately 30% of your total calorie intake. That said, healthy fats such as omega-3 fatty acids are crucial for heart and brain health, controlling blood sugar and cholesterol levels, and reducing chronic inflammation. These can be found in foods like avocados, nuts, seeds, and olive oil.

4. **Fruits and vegetables:** Eating a variety of fruit and vegetables from all colors of the rainbow ensures an adequate intake of vitamins, minerals, fiber, and antioxidants. The minimum recommended intake for fruit and vegetables is 5 portions per day. That could be 3 portions of vegetables and 2 fruits. However, the more you manage to consume, the better for your health, but it is best to focus more on veggies than fruit due to the high sugar content of fruit.

5. **Dairy or dairy alternatives:** Dairy products are a source of protein, carbohydrate, and fat. In addition, they are an excellent source of calcium

for supporting strong bones and teeth. Try to include 2-3 portions of milk, cheese, or yogurt every day. If you prefer, dairy alternatives, look for products such as almond milk that have been fortified with calcium. Nutritionally, soya milk compares favorably with dairy, with the added bonus of having phyto estrogens for managing symptoms of menopause.

In addition to eating a range of foods from all 5 food groups, following a balanced diet also involves limiting your intake of processed foods, sugar, and sodium. While there's nothing like a burger and fries or a sticky dessert to satisfy your food cravings, most of your meals should consist of health foods. To make life more bearable, you can use an 80:20 principle: Eat balanced meals 80% of the time and use the remaining 20% for delectable treats.

Of course, your food intake must be aligned with your calorie requirements. While menopause is often characterized by having an insatiable appetite for all the wrong foods, your energy requirements start to drop. Combined with a stumbling metabolism, it means you need to keep a closer eye on your calorie intake to avoid weight gain.

Last, but not least, hydration is a fundamental part of a balanced diet. Water is found in all parts of your body and all chemical processes that keep you alive need water to take place.

#2. Mediterranean Diet

You may be dreaming of escaping to the Mediterranean for a well-deserved vacation, enjoying a glass of wine under the blue sky overlooking the warm crystal-clear waters of the Mediterranean Sea. While you're there, you can nibble on plump olives and fresh cheese, and feast on the tastiest dishes made only from fresh, locally grown produce. It's the stuff dreams are made of and bound to make the menopause blues evaporate into thin air.

Unfortunately, taking a trip to the Mediterranean is out of reach for most of us, but the food enjoyed by the people of Greece, Italy, and Spain is available worldwide. As a result, everyone can enjoy the health benefits of a Mediterranean inspired diet.

The dietary pattern has been thoroughly studied and has been shown to reduce the risk of chronic diseases such as heart disease, diabetes, and certain types of cancer, including cancer of the breast, colon, cervix, and bladder (Mentella et al., 2019).

According to a study examining the impact of the Mediterranean diet on menopause symptoms, following the eating pattern, in particular, increasing your intake of legumes and olive oil, can significantly reduce your symptoms (Ryczkowska et al., 2022).

The following are the key features of the Mediterranean diet:

1. **Abundance of plant-based foods:** The Mediterranean diet is not a vegan or vegetarian diet, however, there is a strong focus on plant-based foods, including fruits, vegetables, nuts, seeds, wholegrains, and legumes. For this reason, the diet is high in fiber, vitamins, minerals, and antioxidant and anti-inflammatory plant chemicals.

2. **Healthy fats:** Olive oil is the primary form of added fat in the Mediterranean diet. It is used for cooking and dressing salads and is a rich source of healthy monounsaturated fats. Other foods containing healthy fats are also consumed regularly, such as nuts, seeds, and omega-3 rich fatty fish like salmon and sardines.

3. **Fish and poultry:** Fish and poultry are the main types of animal-based protein consumed as part of the Mediterranean diet. They are both low in saturated fat which is good for heart health. In addition, fish is an excellent source of omega-3 fatty acids which reduce the risk of cardiovascular disease and help manage chronic inflammation.

4. **Limited red meat:** When red meat is consumed, it is usually in small portions and used as a flavoring rather than the main focus of a meal. Eating less red meat naturally reduces your intake of saturated fat.

5. **Dairy in moderation:** Traditional Mediterranean diets often include fermented dairy products such as yogurt and cheese, which are a source of beneficial probiotics that promote gut health.

6. **Wine in moderation:** If you're a wine-drinker, this one's for you! Red wine, typically enjoyed in small amounts with meals is thought to contribute to the diet's health benefits due to its antioxidant content. That said, if you don't enjoy red wine, it is only a small part of the Mediterranean diet and not drinking it won't affect the benefits of the meal pattern.

7. **Herbs and spices:** Instead of seasoning food with salt, herbs and spices are used to enhance the flavor. Such ingredients also contribute to the overall nutritional value of the diet.

The Mediterranean diet is about more than just the food you eat. It is a lifestyle that when embraced offers benefits for the body, mind, and soul. As such, daily physical activity, connecting with friends and family, and taking time to enjoy meals can enhance the health-supporting benefits of the diet.

#3. Plant-Based Diet (Vegan/Vegetarian)

Plant-based diets come in several forms depending on whether you choose to eat exclusively plant-based meals, or if you include some animal foods such as eggs and dairy products. Either way, the high intake of nutrient-dense fruits, vegetables, legumes, nuts, seeds, and whole grains are beneficial for overall health.

Following a plant-based diet may also offer relief from the symptoms of menopause. For example, researchers examined the effects of eating a plant-based diet that included a high intake of soybeans. They found that women who consumed more soybeans suffered fewer hot flushes, and experienced better moods, health, and sexual function than women who didn't (Barnard et al., 2021).

Here's a breakdown of both vegan and vegetarian diets:

Vegan diet:

There are no animal products in a vegan diet. That means if you follow a vegan diet, you won't eat any meat, chicken, fish, dairy products, or eggs. You also have to read food labels carefully to ensure that no animal-derived ingredients have been used to make the product. All nutrients are provided by plant-based foods, including fruits, vegetables, legumes (beans, lentils, and chickpeas), whole grains, nuts, seeds, and plant-based oils. Soya products such as tofu, tempeh, and edamame beans are a good source of protein in a vegan diet. Instead of dairy products, people following a vegan diet may choose plant-based milk alternatives. Vegan milk options include almond milk, soy milk, and oat milk, and dairy-free cheeses and yogurt are also available.

Vegetarian diet:

Meat and chicken are generally avoided on a vegetarian diet but animal products such as eggs and dairy products may be allowed.There are several different vegetarian diets, including:

- Lacto-vegetarian: Includes dairy products, but no other animal-based foods.

- Ovo-vegetarian: Includes eggs, but no other animal-based foods.

- Lacto-ovo vegetarian: Includes dairy products and eggs, but no other animal-based foods.

- Pescatarian: Excludes meat and poultry but includes fish and other seafood.

- Flexitarian: This is not strictly a vegetarian diet. It is an eating pattern in which people consume mostly plant-based foods, but occasionally incorporate small amounts of meat and other animal-based products in their meals.

While well-balanced vegan and vegetarian diets are nutrient-dense, there are specific essential nutrients that are found primarily in animal-based foods. As such, it may be necessary to supplement your diet with extra vitamin B12, iron, calcium, and omega-3 fatty acids. It may be useful to consult with a registered dietitian or nutritionist who can help to ensure you eat a well-balanced and healthful plant-based diet.

#4 Low Glycemic Index (GI) Diet

The glycemic index (GI) is a ranking of carbohydrate foods based on the effect they have on your blood sugar levels. Foods that have a dramatic effect on your blood sugar levels are called high GI foods. They are digested quickly, resulting in a rapid rise in blood sugar levels. On the other hand, low GI foods are digested more slowly, releasing glucose into the blood more gradually. They raise blood sugar levels more gradually and more moderately than high GI foods.

When the carbohydrate-containing foods such as grains, fruits, vegetables, and legumes primarily have a low GI, your blood sugar and insulin levels are more stable. Thus a low GI diet is beneficial better blood sugar control, improved insulin sensitivity, sustained energy levels, and easier appetite control.

During menopause, declining estrogen levels cause changes in metabolism. According to research, menopausal women experience higher blood sugar and insulin levels after eating than premenopausal women. It is, therefore, beneficial to consider the glycemic index of the foods you eat to mitigate the increase in blood glucose after a meal (Bermingham et al., 2022).

The basic principles of a low GI diet include:

1. **Choosing low-GI foods:** Complex carbohydrates such as wholegrains, legumes, non-starchy vegetables, and fruits such as berries are excellent choices for a low GI diet. They are typically high in fiber, especially soluble fiber, which slows down digestion, resulting in a gradual and moderate increase in blood sugar levels after a meal.

2. **Balanced meals:** Good blood sugar control involves eating low GI carbohydrates as part of a balanced meal containing protein, fat and vegetables. As an example, your dinner could be a piece of grilled chicken served with a baked sweet potato and a large salad drizzled with olive oil.

3. **Avoiding high-GI foods:** Sugary cereals, white bread, and processed snacks can lead to rapid blood sugar spikes followed by equally rapid

drops. If this happens you may feel tired, irritable, and desperate for something to eat, preferably something sweet that will cause another spike in blood sugar. While your snack may make you feel better, it sets you up for a never ending rollercoaster of blood sugar highs and lows, which ultimately causes weight gain and increases your risk of developing diabetes.

4. **Portion control:** Too much of a good thing can be a problem. In the case of low GI foods, it is crucial to remember that although the carbohydrates are digested slowly, large portions will cause a greater increase in blood sugar.

The glycemic index can be a useful tool for making more informed food choices. However, not all high-GI foods are unhealthy (watermelon), and not all low-GI foods are good for you (ice-cream). It comes down to evaluating the nutrient content of the food you're eating and developing a balanced meal plan that includes foods from all food groups.

#5 DASH Diet

If you have hypertension high blood pressure, you may want to consider the DASH diet. DASH stands for Dietary Approaches to Stop Hypertension. It is an eating plan that was designed by the National Heart, Lung, and Blood Institute (NHLBI) to prevent and control high blood pressure. As such, it is low in sodium (salt) and rich in foods that contain nutrients proven to help manage hypertension such as fruits, vegetables, and low-fat dairy products.

Although the main purpose of the DASH diet is managing blood pressure, due to the types of foods included in the diet, it can also be used to improve overall cardiovascular health and for weight loss.

For women in menopause, the DASH diet has been shown to not only improve heart and bone health, but it may also be beneficial for improving the mood disturbances associated with this stage of life (Torres & Nowson, 2012).

Key features of the DASH diet include:

1. **Low sodium intake:** Salt has been linked to hypertension, and reducing your salt intake can help improve your blood pressure. The maximum amount of sodium included in the DASH diet is 2300mg per day, which is the equivalent of a teaspoon of salt. You can replace salt with herbs, spices, and lemon juice to season your food.

2. **High intake of fruits and vegetables:** Potassium is a critical nutrient for managing blood pressure. Many fruits and vegetables have high levels of potassium, and, therefore, the DASH diet encourages you to

eat a variety of fruits and vegetables, which also provide other essential nutrients, including vitamins, minerals, fiber, and antioxidants.

3. **Whole grains:** Whole grains and other low GI carbohydrates are included in the DASH diet to provide nutrients and a sustained release of energy to keep blood sugar levels within the normal range.

4. **Lean protein:** Red meat is limited on the DASH diet due to its high saturated fat content which is associated with high cholesterol levels. Instead, the diet focuses on leaner protein foods like fish, chicken and legumes.

5. **Dairy:** Low-fat and fat-free dairy products are included for their protein and calcium content. Calcium is as critical for controlling blood pressure as it is for building and maintaining strong bones.

6. **Nuts and seeds:** Nuts and seeds are good sources of omega-3 fatty acids which help to reduce bad cholesterol levels and increase good cholesterol levels. They are also rich in nutrients such as magnesium, calcium, potassium, zinc, and iron.

7. **Limited sweets and added sugars:** Like all healthy diets, sugars and sweets are limited on the DASH diet. Not only are they high in calories, but they also cause a rapid rise in blood sugar levels.

8. **Portion control:** Paying attention to portion sizes encouraged to help manage calorie intake to lose weight and maintain a healthy weight.

The DASH diet is not only for people with high blood pressure. It is suitable for anyone interested in improving the overall quality of their diet and maintaining good heart health.

#6 Anti-Inflammatory Diet

In general, chronic inflammation is associated with several health issues, including heart disease, cancer, autoimmune disorders, and obesity. Pre menopause, estrogen and progesterone protect a woman's body from inflammation, and when hormone levels start to drop, there is a subsequent increase in inflammation. Since menopause is an inflammatory condition, all women in the early stages of perimenopause, those approaching menopause, and those in menopause can benefit from eating more foods containing anti-inflammatory nutrients (McCarthy & Raval, 2020). Scientific studies have shown that menopausal women who eat an anti-inflammatory diet experience better quality of life and less severe menopause symptoms, with significant relief from sexual symptoms such as vaginal dryness and painful sex.

The principles of the anti-inflammatory diet include:

1. **Whole foods:** Whole, minimally processed foods are the cornerstone of an anti-inflammatory diet. Include a variety of fruits, vegetables, whole grains, legumes, nuts, and seeds in your diet every day.

2. **Omega-3 fatty acids:** Omega-3 fatty acids have anti-inflammatory properties. Therefore, eating foods high in healthy fats is advised. Include fatty fish (salmon, trout, sardines), flaxseeds, chia seeds, and walnuts.

3. **Eat the rainbow:** Brightly colored fruits and vegetables, such as strawberries (red), carrots (orange), yellow bell peppers (yellow), broccoli (green), blueberries (blue), and eggplant (purple) are high in antioxidants and phytochemicals (plant chemicals with potent anti-inflammatory properties), which can help combat inflammation.

4. **Dietary fiber:** The fiber found in whole grains, legumes, fruits, and vegetables promotes gut health. It is a source of fuel for the healthy bacteria living in your intestines. They are essential for overall physical and mental health, and produce chemicals that help control inflammation.

5. **Spices and herbs:** Turmeric, ginger, garlic, and cinnamon have anti-inflammatory properties and should be incorporated in an anti-inflammatory diet.

6. **Lean protein:** Saturated fat may promote inflammation. As a result, it is limited in the anti-inflammatory diet and lean sources of protein, including skinless chicken, fish, and legumes are recommended and red meat is restricted.

7. **Limited sugar:** A high intake of refined sugar promotes inflammation. Therefore, sugar intake is limited.

8. **Fermented foods:** Fermented foods contain probiotics which support gut health. To boost your intake of probiotics, choose foods such as yogurt, kefir, kimchi, tempeh, and sauerkraut.

9. **Anti-inflammatory beverages:** Green tea and other herbal teas are rich in antioxidants and consuming them can help fight inflammation. Your choice of beverage can also promote inflammation. Try to avoid sodas, energy drinks, alcohol, sweet coffee drinks, and sweetened teas.

While the anti-inflammatory diet emphasizes foods that may help reduce inflammation, it also encourages a well-balanced approach to eating. The dietary pattern shares many of the same principles of the Mediterranean and DASH diets. It is not a strict plan and it can be customized to suit your personal preferences and dietary needs.

#7 Ketogenic Diet

The keto diet, or ketogenic diet, has become a popular style of eating for people who want to lose weight and body fat. It is a low-carbohydrate, high-fat diet that starves your body of its primary energy source, glucose. When there is not enough sugar in your blood to support your cell's energy requirements, they make a metabolic shift and start burning fat in the form of ketones instead.

When that happens, you are said to be in a state of ketosis. The diet was first used as part of the treatment plan for people with epilepsy, but it has gained recognition for weight loss and its impact on other health conditions such as polycystic ovary syndrome (PCOS), diabetes, and brain disorders.

While the keto diet may seem like the ideal choice for women in menopause due to its blood sugar lowering effect and the improvement in insulin sensitivity often observed in people who follow the diet, there are some drawbacks that cannot be ignored. The most significant risk factor associated with eating a high-fat diet is a rise in blood cholesterol levels. Research shows that levels of both good and bad cholesterol increase, contributing to a higher risk of developing heart disease (Batch et al., 2020).

Therefore, should you feel that the ketogenic diet is the best choice for you, consult with your healthcare practitioner before you begin to avoid these drawbacks.

The key features of the ketogenic diet include:

1. **Low carbohydrate intake:** Carbohydrate intake is severely restricted in the ketogenic diet with only 5-10% of your daily calories coming from carbs. To put this in perspective, it means eating between 20 and 50g of carbohydrates per day mostly in the form of non-starchy vegetables such as spinach, kale, broccoli, cucumber, eggplant, and tomatoes. Depending on your carbohydrate restriction, you may be able to include some quinoa, beans, and lentils in your meal plan, but foods high in carbohydrates like rice, potatoes, and pasta are not included in the keto diet.

2. **High fat intake:** Most of your calories come from fat on the keto diet. You can expect to consume 70-80% of your daily calories in the form of fat. To reduce the risk of high LDL-cholesterol (bad cholesterol), include more healthy fats such as avocados, olive oil, nuts, seeds, and fatty fish in your diet and limit the intake of saturated fats from fatty meat, bacon, and chicken skin.

3. **Moderate protein intake:** Protein can be converted to glucose when there isn't enough carbohydrate in the diet to support your body's energy requirements. As a result, the protein content in the keto diet is moderate, making up 10-20% of your daily calorie intake.

4. **Ketosis:** The primary objective of the ketogenic diet is to achieve and maintain a state of ketosis. In ketosis, fat is converted to ketone bodies in the liver, which serve as an alternative fuel source for the body and brain when carbohydrates are scarce.

5. **Minimized sugar and processed foods:** Foods high in sugar and those that are highly processed, usually cause a spike in blood sugar levels, even in small amounts. Therefore, they are strictly limited in the keto diet. As soon as your blood sugar rises, your cells switch back to burning glucose for energy instead of ketones, thus inhibiting ketosis.

6. **Whole foods:** While the diet is often associated with unhealthy high-fat foods like butter and bacon, many ketogenic diet supporters advocate for the inclusion of whole, nutrient-dense foods like non-starchy vegetables, grass-fed meat, fatty fish, eggs, and dairy products (if tolerated).

The ketogenic diet is a specialized and restrictive diet that is not suitable for everyone. The best versions of the diet focus on eating whole foods, including lean meat, fish, eggs, non-starchy vegetables, and healthy fats. However, the diet can lead to a range of side effects, including the "keto flu" (flu-like symptoms that some people experience when they first enter ketosis), electrolyte imbalances, constipation, and potential increases in cholesterol levels. Moreover, the long-term implications of following the diet are still being researched, and it may not be recommended for individuals with certain medical conditions. Consult with your doctor or healthcare provider before starting the ketogenic diet.

#8 Macrobiotic Diet

Originating in Japan, the macrobiotic diet is a lifestyle approach based on the principles of Zen Buddhism and traditional Japanese eating patterns. The main purpose of the combined lifestyle practices is to create balance between the different elements to achieve harmony within the body.

There is a strong focus on eating whole plant-based foods that are seasonal, organic, and locally sourced. While the emphasis is on plant-based foods, some forms of the diet allow small amounts of lean meat and fish.

The diet has been extensively researched for its benefits in aiding with the treatment and prevention of breast cancer. However, the type of food included in the diet, makes it a good choice for people with heart disease and diabetes too (Soare et al., 2016).

Use the principles below to follow the macrobiotic diet:

1. **Whole foods:** Eat mostly whole, minimally processed foods like whole grains, beans, legumes, vegetables, fruits, seeds, and nuts.

2. **Balance of yin and yang:** The cornerstone of the macrobiotic philosophy is achieving a balance between the yin and yang qualities in food to create harmony in the body. Yin foods include fruits and leafy green vegetables and are considered more expansive and cooling. On the other hand, yang foods like grains and root vegetables are seen as more contractive and warming.

3. **Local and seasonal foods:** The practice of eating food that is in season and locally grown not only boosts your nutrient intake, but it is also believed to be in harmony with nature and the environment.

4. **Whole grains:** Brown rice and other whole grains are a staple of the macrobiotic diet. They are considered to be a balanced source of nutrition and provide energy for the body.

5. **Vegetables:** There is a strong focus on including a wide variety of vegetables in the macrobiotic diet. Leafy greens, root vegetables, and sea vegetables (like seaweed), form a large proportion of your food intake.

6. **Protein sources:** While some variations of the diet allow small amounts of fish to be included in the diet, plant-based proteins form the bulk of your protein intake. They include beans, lentils, chickpeas, tofu, and tempeh.

7. **Cooking methods:** There is an emphasis on simple and gently cooking methods when you follow the macrobiotic diet. Most meals are cooked by steaming, blanching, or quickly sautéing food.

8. **Mindful eating:** One of the lifestyle aspects of the macrobiotic diet is mindful eating practices. You are encouraged to take your time over meals, be fully present while savoring each mouthful.

The macrobiotic diet is not just about what you eat but also about how you eat, and it encourages a holistic approach to health and well-being. However, the macrobiotic diet is a restrictive eating pattern and may not provide all essential nutrients, particularly if followed in its strictest form. Similar to following other plant-based diets, you may need to consider supplementing your intake with vitamin B12, calcium, and iron.

Which Diet is the Best Choice for You?

You will have noticed when reading through the characteristics of each diet that they all have some critical elements in common. For example, all 8 diets encourage you to eat whole foods that have been minimally processed and to avoid highly processed foods that are typically high in sugar and processed fats and calories. They all also promote the intake of plenty of vegetables and some fruits in as many colors as you can find.

The inflammatory nature of menopause means your body becomes more susceptible to the adverse effects of stress. Diets that eliminate specific foods groups or rely on a very low-calorie intake, can increase the amount of stress your body has to manage and increase your risk for chronic disease.

Use your inner wisdom as a menopausal woman to make informed choices about the food you eat to promote good health and potentially improve the symptoms that characterize this time of your life.

INTERMITTENT FASTING AND DETOX DIETS – PROS AND CONS

Y our jeans are getting tighter by the day, and yet you seem to have no control over what or how much you eat. The number on the scale keeps climbing, and your weight is the highest it has ever been. Despite following a healthy diet and going to the gym every day, you are feeling uncomfortable in your own skin, and you have started wondering if you must resign yourself to the dreaded "middle-age spread."

The changes your body undergoes during midlife can be frustrating. Altered metabolism and inflammation because of declining levels of reproductive hormones, combined with a voracious appetite, seem to make weight gain unavoidable. Apart from your expanding waistline, your doctor has also started talking to you about chronic diseases and how following a healthy diet can help manage such conditions. All the same, even though you are eating a healthy, balanced diet, drinking plenty of water, and exercising daily, you are not making any progress.

Are there any alternatives or additional dietary approaches to kickstart your weight loss and boost your metabolism? In desperation, you may be tempted to turn to scientifically unproven, nutritionally unbalanced fad diets in an effort to shift your weight. While you may initially experience dramatic weight loss, your success is usually short-lived and the weight you lost returns, often bringing friends along with it, leaving you heavier than before you started. As such, diets that promise dramatic results with little effort are usually too good to be true.

In this chapter, we will explore the pros and cons of popular eating styles and weight loss methods including intermittent fasting and detox diets. The benefits and drawbacks of each one will be evaluated, arming you with the information you need to make informed decisions about which option is best suited to your health and weight loss needs.

Intermittent Fasting

First on the list is intermittent fasting. It has grown in popularity in recent years as a dietary strategy that promotes both weight loss and improved health. Although there are several methods of intermittent fasting, they all involve not eating or restricting your calorie intake for a period of time while eating normally during your eating window.

Fasting is not a new concept. It has been an important part of many religions and cultures for thousands of years. However, the dietary practice has only recently been recognized for its potential benefits for health and weight management. Furthermore, research shows that intermittent fasting may be useful for women's health in both pre- and post-menopause (Nair & Khawale, 2016).

Benefits and Drawbacks of Intermittent Fasting

Some of the benefits of intermittent fasting during menopause include the following:

- **Weight management:** Research suggests that intermittent fasting can contribute to weight loss. The eating style helps your body burn fat more efficiently while maintaining lean muscle mass. Studies also show that intermittent fasting is an effective weight loss tool for women of all ages, both pre- and post-menopause (Lin et al., 2021).

- **Improved insulin sensitivity:** Intermittent fasting may improve insulin sensitivity, which is particularly relevant during menopause when insulin resistance can contribute to weight gain and raised blood sugar levels (Vasim et al., 2022).

- **Appetite regulation:** Although some women may feel hungrier than usual when they practice intermittent fasting, it can have the opposite effect. Some research suggests that fasting may influence hormone levels, such as insulin, leptin, and ghrelin, which regulate your metabolism and appetite (Oliveira et al., 2022).

- **Reduced inflammation:** Declining levels of sex hormones result in increased inflammation in the body. Intermittent fasting may have an anti-inflammatory effect, helping to reduce the risk of chronic diseases such as diabetes and heart disease. However, study results are mixed, and further research needs to be done to confirm this potential benefit of fasting (Jordan et al., 2019).

- **Cellular repair and longevity:** Some forms of intermittent fasting may induce autophagy, a biological housekeeping process that destroys and removes dead cells throughout the body. Research suggests that it offers potential anti-aging benefits. Unfortunately, as women age and estrogen levels drop, this beneficial process diminishes. However, studies show that fasting can restore the body's ability to self-clean, thus improving health and longevity (Shabkhizan et al., 2023).

As appealing as the benefits of intermittent fasting are, the drawbacks must also be considered before deciding to include the practice in your dietary regime. For one thing, there are concerns that intermittent fasting might further affect hormonal balance, potentially exacerbating menopausal symptoms. Although scientific studies have shown that fasting has little to no impact on estrogen levels, it may result in a drop in testosterone levels (Cienfuegos et al., 2022).

Another concern about the safety of intermittent fasting is nutritional deficiencies. Since a balanced diet is crucial for ensuring your health and well-being during menopause, and the amounts of some nutrients such as calcium are increased at this time of your life, it is critical to ensure that you are eating a balanced diet that meets your body's requirements when practicing any form of fasting.

In addition, women who have a history of disordered eating like anorexia, bulimia, or binge-eating disorder should avoid intermittent fasting as it may trigger the condition. Furthermore, some studies reveal that this dietary style may increase the risk of mood disorders, including depression, anxiety, and irritability.

Finally, intermittent fasting may increase hunger and food cravings, cause brain fog, and a drop in energy levels (Harvie & Howell, 2017).

Once you have weighed up the pros and cons of intermittent fasting, you must choose a method that fits your lifestyle and daily routines while meeting your body's need for energy and nutrients. There are several forms of fasting, ranging from 24-hour fasts to alternate-day fasting and time-restricted eating (Nowosad & Sujka, 2021). The three methods of intermittent fasting that work best for most people are described in the next section.

Types of Intermittent Fasting

16/8 Method

The 16/8 method of intermittent fasting is a form of time-restricted eating. It involves fasting for 16 hours and restricting eating to an 8-hour window each day during which you eat a healthy balanced diet. Many people find this method easy to include in their daily routine, but some find it challenging to not eat for as long as 16 hours. To increase your chances of success, it is best to start slowly. Begin with a 12-hour fast and 12-hour eating window and increase your fasting over a few weeks until you feel comfortable with the 16/8 split.

Eat-Stop-Eat

The Eat-Stop-Eat method involves a 24-hour fast once or twice a week. For example, it means eating dinner and then not eating or restricting your calorie intake until the next evening. This method is effective for weight loss, but the 24-hour fasting period can be difficult for some people. To make it easier to fast for 24 hours, drink plenty of water, unsweetened tea and coffee, or other non-caloric drinks during your fast and ensure your meal is high in protein and fiber to keep you feeling fuller for longer.

5:2 Diet

When you embrace the 5:2 diet you eat normally for five days of the week and consume a very low calorie (around 500-600 calories) diet on the remaining two non-consecutive days. For example, you may choose to fast on Monday and Thursday every week. This fasting method is flexible as you can change your fasting days depending on your schedule. If you have to go to a work function on your usual fasting day, for instance, you can simply fast the day before or after instead. However, the low-calorie intake on fasting days can be challenging for some people.

Intermittent fasting during menopause can offer potential benefits for weight management and metabolic health, but it should be approached with caution. The choice of the fasting method must be based on your unique preferences, lifestyle, and health considerations. For best results and to ensure your health and well-being, you should consult with your healthcare practitioner or a registered dietitian to ensure that your intermittent fasting regimen of choice is safe, balanced, and meets your nutritional needs during this life stage.

Detox Diets

Detox diets are often promoted as a means of eliminating toxins from the body and improving overall health, usually involving a period of fasting followed by a strict diet of fruits, vegetables, juices, and water. They also typically promise rapid and dramatic weight loss results. Younger women may be able to follow such strict dietary regimes, bouncing back when they return to their normal eating habits. However, during menopause, extreme energy restriction and eliminating entire food groups, even for a few days, can be taxing on your body.

When considering a detox diet during menopause, it's essential to review the potential benefits and drawbacks of such dietary restrictions. Below is an overview of the pros and cons of detox diets during menopause, with a focus on various types such as juice cleanses, smoothie or shake detoxes, tea detox, raw or whole food detox, and supplement-based detoxes.

Benefits and Drawbacks of Detox Diets

Below is a list of potential benefits of following a detox diet:

- **Nutrient Boost:** Some detox diets emphasize the consumption of nutrient-dense, whole foods like fruit and vegetables, providing essential vitamins and minerals that support overall health, including bone health during menopause.

- **Hydration:** Juice cleanses, and smoothie detoxes typically include foods like fruit and vegetables with a high water content. They are also often blended with water, thus promoting hydration, which is crucial during menopause to alleviate symptoms like hot flashes and maintain overall health.

- **Weight Management:** Detox diets may lead to short-term weight loss due to caloric restriction, which can be appealing to women experiencing weight gain during menopause.

- **Increased Fruit and Vegetable Intake:** Many detox diets encourage the consumption of fruits and vegetables, rich in vitamins, minerals, and fiber, which are good for overall health.

The allure of the promises made by those promoting detox diets can be difficult to resist, especially when you are trying to manage the symptoms of menopause. The frustration of not losing weight can make a detox diet seem like your knight in shining weight loss armor. Unfortunately, such diets seldom provide enough energy and nutrients to support your body, and if followed for more than a few days, can result in nutritional deficiencies and muscle loss(Tahreem et al., 2022).

Detox diets are usually very restrictive, making them difficult to follow for more than two to three days. Another problem is that the extreme energy restriction may result in rapid weight loss, but it is not sustainable. This is because water is stored along with every molecule of sugar that is stored in your muscles and liver. When you are not eating enough calories, your body uses up all your energy reserves, releasing the water and resulting in weight loss. As soon as you start eating normally again, your energy reserves are restored, and the number on the scale increases again (Fernández-Elías et al., 2015).

The biggest concern about detox diets is that their claims are typically not backed by scientific evidence. While an increase in certain nutrients may help support your body's built in detox processes, your liver, kidneys, and digestive system continue to remove toxic substances and waste products from your body regardless of what you eat (Tahreem et al., 2022).

Types of Detox Diets

Juice Cleanses

A juice cleanse involves drinking only fresh fruit and vegetable juices for a specified number of days. Depending on the cleanse you choose, you may be encouraged to drink only fresh juices. However, some versions of a juice cleanse allow you to eat whole fruit, steamed vegetables, and plain boiled or steamed potatoes. Consuming only fresh fruit and vegetable juices increases your intake of vitamins. Still, such a diet lacks essential nutrients like protein and may lead to blood sugar fluctuations (Henning et al., 2017).

Smoothie or Shake Detoxes

Smoothies made from fruits, vegetables, and protein sources such as nuts or shakes made from formulated meal replacement powders are sometimes promoted as a form of detox diet. Liquid meals like these can be convenient and nutrient-dense but may lack fiber and essential nutrients. Smoothies can also have a high sugar content if care is not taken to control how much fruit or fruit juice is used to make them.

Tea Detox

Detox teas include a variety of herbal ingredients like Guarana, cinnamon, red clover, ginger root, and burdock root. A tea detox involves consuming herbal teas or special detox teas to boost your body's detoxification processes. Some teas contain potent antioxidants, but their detoxifying effects are often overstated. Drinking some detox teas in large amounts can have side effects like nausea and diarrhea and, in extreme cases, can cause liver failure (Kesavarapu et al., 2017).

Raw or Whole Food Detox

The diet emphasizes the intake of raw, unprocessed foods such as fruits, vegetables, and nuts. Consuming such foods helps eliminate artificial food additives and preservatives from your diet. A raw or whole foods diet is usually rich in essential nutrients. However, it may be challenging to maintain and could lead to nutrient imbalances if you do not ensure a balanced intake of carbohydrates, protein, and fat (Abraham et al., 2022).

Supplement-Based Detoxes

Some detox programs involve taking supplements or special products that claim to aid in detoxification. Such products include activated charcoal, spirulina, and a variety of vitamins and minerals like iron and vitamin B2 (Tinsley et al., 2018). There is little scientific evidence to support the use of detox supplements.

Detox diets may offer some benefits, such as increased nutrient intake and hydration, but they also come with potential drawbacks, including nutrient deficiencies and unsustainability. Before embarking on any detox diet, especially during menopause, it's crucial to consult with your healthcare professional or registered dietitian to ensure that the diet you choose is safe, balanced, and meets your specific health needs during midlife. Additionally, focusing on long-term, sustainable dietary changes may be more beneficial for overall health and well-being during and after menopause.

Instead of following a strict detox diet, there are several lifestyle habits that naturally support your body's detoxification processes. They include limiting your intake of alcohol and refined, sugary foods, getting enough good quality sleep, drinking plenty of water, and eating foods rich in antioxidants such as brightly colored fruit and vegetables.

Safety First

Your health and well-being are a priority no matter how old you are. During menopause, though, eating a nutritionally balanced diet that meets your changing energy and nutrient needs becomes critical for supporting your body through the midlife transition. Therefore, rather than choosing a dietary regime based only on its potential to help you shed a few extra pounds, select one that will not contribute to discomfort and irrational moods.

Intermittent fasting combined with a healthy diet offers several health and weight loss benefits, and it is safe for most women to follow. On the other hand, detox diets may do more harm than good. If you are uncertain of which diet is best for you, consult with a nutrition professional who can guide you in choosing a diet that meets your unique needs.

Benefits of Exercise and Physical Activity for Menopause

From unwanted weight gain to age-related muscle loss, menopause is a challenging transition for many women. When you are struggling to get a good night's sleep due to night sweats and you are experiencing fatigue as a result of dropping hormone levels, the last thing you feel like doing is exercising. However, exercise is a powerful ally amidst the array of changes occurring in your body, offering not just physical benefits but also contributing significantly to emotional and mental well-being. In this chapter, we explore the importance of exercise during menopause, discuss the types of exercises that prove most beneficial for women in midlife, and provide practical insights on establishing a sustainable exercise routine.

Importance of Exercise During Menopause

There is no reason to limp through the menopausal transition, hoping you will feel better once your periods stop for good. One way to make the journey easier is to build regular physical activity into your routine. It can make the middle years of your life more bearable, both physically and mentally (Mishra et al., 2011).

One of the greatest benefits of exercise is the role it plays in supporting cardiovascular health. As you are aware, declining hormone levels cause changes to your metabolism and how your body processes fat and sugar, resulting in chronic health conditions such as diabetes and high blood pressure. Regular exercise that gets your heart pumping faster offers protection from these issues by improving how sugar is used by your cells, reducing harmful cholesterol levels, and strengthening your cardiovascular system, thereby reducing the risk of raised blood pressure, heart attacks, and strokes.

Exercise is also beneficial for weight loss. When you move your body, it makes you breathe harder, your heart beat faster, and your cells burn more energy. Therefore, regular physical activity creates an energy deficit that may help support weight loss, even during menopause.

In addition, since bone loss is a consequence of a drop in estrogen levels, it is critical to support bone health however you can. Weight-bearing exercises such as lifting weights or activities that cause an impact on the bones and joints, like walking and jogging, not only support the maintenance of muscle mass but also help keep your bones strong and healthy.

One of the most notable benefits of exercise during menopause is the positive effect it has on mood. Endorphins, often referred to as "feel-good" hormones, are released during exercise, helping alleviate stress, anxiety, and depression that can accompany hormonal changes.

Finally, some women report that exercise helps to manage other symptoms of menopause, including night sweats and hot flashes. It can also help improve your energy levels and improve your sleep.

Adding exercise to your daily routine can feel overwhelming when you already have a lot on your plate. However, it is an essential form of self-care. Remember that any activity that increases your heart rate offers healthy benefits. As such, you can choose a form of exercise you enjoy, be it a cardio workout at the gym or a gentle stroll in the park with your dog. Whatever you do, though, start slowly and build up the intensity of your exercise. Being over-ambitious at the beginning of a new exercise routine can set you up for failure. Instead, ensure success by choosing an activity you enjoy, one you can do with a friend, and starting at a pace or intensity that is manageable for your fitness level.

Types of Exercises Beneficial for Menopausal Women

Though all movement is good for your health, some forms of exercise promote your well-being better than others, whether you are premenopausal, going through perimenopause, or in menopause. For instance, cardiovascular exercise, strength training, and flexibility workouts each work your body differently, offering unique benefits, as explained below. The best exercise routine incorporates workouts from each category to support heart, bone, muscle, and brain health in midlife.

Cardiovascular exercises

Aerobic or cardiovascular exercise is a cornerstone of a menopause exercise routine. Activities such as brisk walking, jogging, swimming, and cycling get the heart pumping and improve overall cardiovascular health. General exercise guidelines recommend that you aim for at least 150 minutes of moderate-intensity aerobic exercise per week (Mishra et al., 2011). You can judge the intensity of your exercise by your breathing rate and how comfortable it is to have a conversation with your exercise buddy. For example, when you are working out at a moderate intensity, your heart will beat faster, and you will breathe harder, but you will still be able to talk, but singing will be difficult.

Not only does this help manage weight by boosting your metabolism and burning more calories, but it also enhances your energy levels and improves your sleep quality. What's more, you can experience these effects through 30 minutes of daily exercise. You do not even have to do it all in a single session. For example, you can go for a brisk 10-minute walk in the morning, climb the stairs at the office, and finish your day with some gardening. Every little exercise that gets your heart pumping counts towards your daily total.

Strength training

As estrogen levels decline, women may experience a loss of bone density and muscle mass. Strength training, involving activities like weightlifting or resistance exercises, becomes crucial in countering these effects. Not only does it enhance muscle strength and tone, but it also helps prevent osteoporosis by promoting bone health. Engage in strength training exercises at least twice a week, targeting the major muscle groups of your legs, abdomen, back, and arms (Mishra et al., 2011).

Don't worry if the first thing you think of when you read "strength training" is young women at the gym wearing tights and a crop top, carrying a water bottle as they move from one fancy weight machine to the next. If that doesn't appeal to you, there are other ways to incorporate strength training into your exercise routine. You can easily build muscle strength at home using your body weight to add resistance to your movements by doing exercises such as squats and pushups. Alternatively, you could invest in free weights like dumbbells or resistance bands and perform exercises like bicep curls, bent-over rows, and bench presses. Always ensure that your technique is correct to avoid injury. Ask an exercise professional, such as a biokineticist, for advice before you start a new strength training program.

Flexibility and balance exercises

The third aspect of an effective exercise routine in midlife is a movement that helps alleviate the joint stiffness and poor balance that become more common as women age and hormone levels drop. As such, exercises that stretch the muscles and gently move the joints help improve your mobility. The workouts that keep your body flexible involve controlled movements and engage your abdominal muscles, which are critical for good posture and balance.

Therefore, incorporating flexibility exercises such as yoga or Pilates into your weekly routine can improve joint mobility and alleviate discomfort. Additionally, balance exercises, like Tai Chi, help reduce the risk of falls, which can become more prevalent with age. Integrating these exercises into your routine improves overall physical well-being (Mishra et al., 2011).

An added benefit of Yoga, Pilates, and Tai Chi is the focus on your breath. The movements are slow and controlled, and your breathing forms part of each exercise, posture, or movement, making such workouts a form of meditation. As you will see in the next chapter, taking time out of your busy day to let go of your responsibilities and turn your attention inward is a useful way to reduce stress and improve your mood.

Developing a sustainable exercise routine

It is never too late to start exercising. Considering that the health effects of a sedentary lifestyle have been compared to those of smoking cigarettes, putting on some comfy clothes and lacing up your sneakers has the potential to add some years to your life. While this may be an exaggeration of the results of scientific research, those who are not active for the recommended 30 minutes per day are more likely to die sooner than those who enjoy daily exercise (Vallance et al., 2018).

Embarking on an exercise routine during menopause requires a thoughtful approach for long-term success. Begin gradually, especially if you've been inactive, and consult with a healthcare professional before starting a new exercise program. Use the tips below to get you started and help you stick with your new exercise program.

10 Tips to help you develop an exercise routine:

1. **Choose a form of exercise you enjoy.** Remember, all physical activity that raises your heart rate and makes you breathe harder counts as exercise. Therefore, you can choose a more formal approach by doing workouts such as swimming, cycling, jogging, or going to the gym, or

you can engage in something you find more pleasurable, like dancing, gardening, or hiking. Remember that your joints are not as flexible as they once were. Therefore, if your goal is to start jogging, for example, begin with walking, building up your strength and stamina over time before exposing your ankles, knees, and hips to the impact of jogging or running.

2. **Start slowly.** It can be tempting to jump in and start working out at a high intensity. Unfortunately, it takes a little time to build up your fitness level. By starting at a slower pace or lesser intensity, you will gradually improve your muscle mass and your cardiovascular fitness. Then, you can start pushing yourself a little harder to increase your fitness even more.

3. **Make it a sociable activity.** You don't have to push yourself through a workout on your own. Making a plan to exercise with a friend or a group of women adds an element of fun and relaxation to your exercise routine. It also makes you accountable to someone else, reducing the risk of making excuses not to exercise.

4. **Use music to make it more pleasurable:** Exercise can feel like hard work. Doing your workout to your favorite tunes can make it much more fun and put an extra bounce in your step.

5. **Book an appointment with yourself.** Put your exercise in your diary so you cannot book anything else in the time slot you have designated to improve your physical and mental well-being. It may not be a fool-proof way of making you move your body, but it is at least a reminder that you must do so.

6. **Mix it up.** While cardiovascular exercise is essential for good health, strength training builds strong muscles and bones, and flexibility and balance workouts keep you supple and help prevent falls as you age.

7. **Be consistent:** There will be days when exercising can make you feel exhausted. That's okay. Skip a day if necessary and pick up your routine the next day. It is also useful to do a gentler workout, such as a stroll around the park when you don't feel up to more intense exercise. It will make it easier to stick with your new routine in the long run.

8. **Be flexible:** Similar to what was mentioned above, it is critical to listen to your body. For example, if you are having a day where you are experiencing heart palpitations and feeling fatigued, exercise could make you feel worse.

9. **Be kind to yourself:** Midlife is a time to practice self-care. Instead of

beating yourself up when the busyness of life gets in the way of your exercise routine, forgive yourself and move on. Tomorrow is another day.

10. **Celebrate your success:** Celebrate your victories no matter how big or small. If you are new to exercise and did three complete pushups for the first time, that is a win. So is running your first five-mile race and swimming ten laps of the pool.

In conclusion, exercise is a powerful tool for managing the challenges of menopause. By incorporating a diverse range of activities, you can not only alleviate your symptoms but also enhance your overall well-being, making this chapter of life a time of empowerment and positive transformation.

Impact of Menopause on Mental Health and Self-Esteem

O *ne of the first signs of perimenopause for Linda was "meno rage". As a 45-year-old divorced stay-at-home mother of three teenage boys with aging parents, Linda has very little time to focus on her own well-being. Not only does she have to manage her sons' teen moodiness, but she must also help her mom and dad with with their daily tasks. She used to be the one who was always calm and in control of every situation, but when her estrogen levels started dropping, she began losing her temper every time one of her sons did something that irritated her. She knew her reaction was irrational and exaggerated, even while she was yelling, but she had no control over her anger. Moreover, when she wasn't yelling, she was feeling down, and tears would roll down her cheeks for no reason at all. She confided in her best friend that it felt like she was losing her mind because she had no control over her emotions. She suggested that Linda talk to her doctor to help her find a solution to her mental health issues. After a thorough investigation that included a medical history and a discussion of Linda's symptoms, combined with several blood tests, the doctor concluded that Linda was going through the menopausal transition. She gave Linda advice on how to manage it and rediscover the person she used to be.*

Mental Health During Menopause

When people talk about menopause, they will often joke about women having hot flashes and commiserate about their inability to get a good night's sleep. Yet, the mental health impact of menopause is typically ignored. It may be because midlife is characterized by high-pressure work environments as women progress in their careers, along with more demands on their time from their growing children and aging parents. Like, Linda, it is also a time when your relationship with your partner changes, sometimes ending in divorce. These external factors are enough to cause depression and anxiety. However, the changes taking place in your body also contribute to these mood disruptions.

While menopause is primarily associated with physical changes, such as the end of your menstrual periods and dry skin, it can also have a significant impact on your mental health. For instance, a decline in the production of hormones like estrogen and progesterone can contribute to mood swings, irritability, and anxiety. That's because estrogen plays a role in regulating neurotransmitters like serotonin and norepinephrine, which are associated with mood regulation. Therefore, the decline in estrogen levels during menopause can disrupt the delicate balance of these neurotransmitters, potentially leading to changes in mood (Barth et al., 2015).

Consequently, as many as one in four women may experience symptoms of depression and anxiety during menopause. The hormonal changes that define this time in a woman's life, combined with factors such as sleep disturbances and high levels of stress, can contribute to low mood and anxiety. Moreover, if you have a history of depression or anxiety, you may be more susceptible to experiencing depressive symptoms during menopause, and they may become worse than they were when you were younger (El Khoudary et al., 2019).

Mood Swings

Like Linda, it is common for women to experience mood swings during menopause. One minute, you are feeling happy and carefree, and the next, you are angry and irritable. It can be exhausting feeling as if you have no control over your mood. While you may be faced with several challenges in your forties and fifties, external factors are not solely to blame. While fluctuating hormones may cause depression and anxiety, they can also make you more irritable.

Note that not all women battle with unpredictable moods as they transition to menopause. Also, the frequency and intensity of these mood disruptions typically varies between women and individuals. In other words, some women may experience mild and occasional mood fluctuations, while others may find their moods swinging more dramatically and often. That is because there are several factors that affect the intensity of mood swings like genetics, lifestyle, and overall health (El Khoudary et al., 2019).

Although declining hormone levels are largely to blame for your moodiness, it helps to figure out what triggers your dramatic mood swings. Are you feeling stressed? Are you getting enough sleep? Or are you dealing with several personal or professional challenges? It is easier to manage your mood swings when you know what is causing them. For example, if you are feeling tired all the time and snapping at your spouse and your children, it may help to seek advice on how to get a better night's sleep. On the other hand, if you are under pressure at work, learning better stress management techniques (to be discussed later in this chapter), such as meditation and deep breathing, can help you cope better overall.

Mood swings can have a significant impact on relationships, both personally and professionally. Therefore, it is crucial for women experiencing menopausal mood swings to communicate openly with their partners, family members, and colleagues. When the people in your life understand you are not being unreasonable simply for the sake of being difficult, they are more likely to treat you with kindness and understanding.

If your mood swings become severe and are affecting your daily life, it is essential to seek professional help. Mental health professionals, such as therapists or counselors, can provide support and guidance in developing coping strategies and addressing underlying emotional concerns.

Next time you feel the anger rising from your belly and erupting from your mouth, remember that mood swings are a common challenge for women in midlife. Understanding the hormonal changes and external factors that contribute to these fluctuations and identifying your triggers, makes it possible to implement coping strategies that can help you navigate this aspect of the menopausal journey more effectively. Seeking support from healthcare professionals, as well as friends and family, is an important step in managing mood swings and promoting overall emotional well-being during this transitional phase of life.

Memory Problems and Difficulty Concentrating

Have you been experiencing *brain fog* as you get closer to your fiftieth birthday? If you have been walking into a room and forgetting why you're there or struggling to find words when you're telling a story, then, your brain is probably suffering from the effects of dropping hormone levels.

The official name is impaired cognitive function which means that your brain is not working as well as it used to. It is not a problem for all women during menopause, but it affects up to 62%. Research shows that the parts of the brain responsible for verbal memory and executive function are most sensitive to fluctuations in female sex hormones. As a result, it changes in your ability to focus and follow directions. In addition, these brain alterations also contribute to your mood swings and changes in self-control (Conde et al., 2021).

Impaired cognitive function is characterized by the following factors:

1. **Memory changes:** Declining hormone levels can cause changes in memory that include forgetfulness and difficulty retaining or recalling information. Such memory lapses can be frustrating and may have an impact on daily activities, such as remembering appointments or peo-

ple's names.

2. **Attention and concentration:** Menopause-related cognitive changes can also affect attention and concentration. Some women report feeling easily distracted or having difficulty staying focused on tasks. This can make staying on top of your work and personal responsibilities challenging, affecting your productivity.

3. **Processing speed:** Cognitive processing speed is the ability to process information quickly and efficiently. This is also influenced by female sex hormones and may be affected during menopause. You may find that tasks you were once able to complete quickly and with ease now take longer or require more effort.

4. **Executive function:** Executive functions, including problem-solving, decision-making, and planning, may be influenced by hormonal changes, making managing daily responsibilities more challenging.

Impaired cognitive function during menopause is a multifaceted and complex phenomenon. If cognitive changes during menopause are causing you distress or affecting your daily life, you must consult with your healthcare professional. Their assessment of your brain function may involve cognitive assessments and discussions about your overall health and well-being. Your doctor will give you advice about what you can do to support your brain health such as eating a healthy diet, being physically active, and getting enough good quality sleep etc.

Menopause and Body Image and Self-Esteem

In modern society, women are expected to be slender with flawless skin and shiny hair. However, women come in all shapes and sizes and their appearance is determined by the genes they inherited from their parents as well as health conditions and their lifestyle habits. As a result, many women struggle to cultivate a positive body image throughout their lives.

Your body image is a concept including factors such as how you perceive your body, your thoughts about your appearance, and how you feel about the way you appear to others. While some women embrace their bodies no matter how they look, many are self-conscious about their physical appearance and may worry that their bodies don't look or work the same way as other women. Then, when you enter your forties and fifties, menopause and the associated signs and symptoms cause changes to your body's structure and function, potentially resulting in further body-image issues.

Dissatisfaction with your changing body shape during menopause can have a profound influence on your mental health. You may even feel a sense of loss related to your youthful appearance, affecting how you see yourself in the mirror.

When your changing hormone levels result in weight gain around your belly and smaller, weaker muscles, not to mention less elastic, wrinkled skin, and thinning hair, it can be difficult to come to terms with your new appearance. Furthermore, hot flashes and night sweats can make you feel uncomfortable in your own skin, further affecting your body image.

In addition to this, the resulting changes of declining hormone levels in your vagina can have a significant impact on your desire for intimacy. Not only does estrogen influence the blood flow to the genitourinary system resulting in less desire to engage in sexual intercourse, but vaginal dryness may cause discomfort during intimacy, further reducing your confidence in your body. On the other hand, a poor self-image and feeling down about your body can also reduce your sexual appetite.

A combination of a negative self-image with less desire for intimacy and an array of menopausal symptoms may result in poor self-esteem. Also, the middle years of your life are characterized by important life changes such as your children growing up and leaving home and shifts in your career. Consequently, it is a time in your life when you may begin reevaluating your self-worth and life's purpose, potentially redefining your identity and the roles you play in society (Vincent et al., 2023).

As such, the menopausal transition can also be an opportunity for cultivating a positive body image and boosting your self-esteem. When you embrace the changes as a natural part of life and focus on the wisdom and experiences that come with age, it becomes possible to adopt a positive mindset and practice self-compassion, thus promoting overall well-being. Finally, engaging in self-care practices that promote overall well-being can positively impact body image. This includes regular exercise, a balanced diet, and activities that bring joy and relaxation. Taking care of the body in a holistic manner can contribute to a more positive self-esteem.

In the following section, we will explore proven ways to boost your mental health and develop a healthy body image and positive self-esteem during menopause. From lifestyle changes to mindfulness practices, and cognitive behavioral therapy, there is a strategy that will help you overcome the mental challenges associated with midlife.

12 Strategies for Improved Mental Health During Menopause

The World Health Organization (WHO) defines health as "a state of complete physical, mental, and social well-being and not merely the absence of disease of infirmity" (*Constitution of the World Health Organization*, n.d.). Therefore, while physical health is critical for your well-being, your mental health cannot be ignored.

Use the twelve strategies listed below to improve and support your mental health during menopause:

1. **Regular physical activity:** Engaging in regular exercise has been shown to have numerous benefits for mental health. Exercise can help alleviate stress, improve mood, and boost overall well-being (Smith & Merwin, 2021).

2. **Healthy diet:** Eating a nutritious and balanced diet is essential for supporting both physical and mental health. Include a variety of fruits, vegetables, whole grains, lean proteins, and healthy fats in your meal plan (refer to Chapter 7 for more details).

3. **Adequate sleep:** It may be difficult to get a good night's sleep when your hormone levels change, but prioritizing sleep is crucial for mental health and cognitive function. Sleep hygiene strategies can help ensure that you get enough good quality sleep. Some examples of good sleep hygiene include going to bed and waking up at the same time every day, ensuring your sleep environment is comfortable, and practicing relaxation techniques before bedtime (Scott et al., 2021).

4. **Stress management:** Stress management techniques can help you cope with the challenges of menopause. Practices such as mindfulness meditation, deep breathing exercises, progressive muscle relaxation, or engaging in activities that bring joy and relaxation can reduce your stress levels and improve your mood (Worthen, n.d.).

5. **Social support:** A sense of belonging has been proven to prevent and manage mental health issues. Being able to share your experiences with other people, whether they are friends, family, or coworkers, makes it easier to cope when life gets tough. Connecting with people can help you manage stress, anxiety, and depression (*How Does Social Connectedness Affect Health?* | *CDC*, 2023).

6. **Counseling or therapy:** Seeking the guidance of a mental health professional, such as a counselor or therapist, can offer valuable support. Therapy can provide a safe space to explore and navigate the emotional aspects of menopause, offering coping strategies and tools such as cognitive behavioral therapy (discussed later) for managing stress.

7. **Mindfulness and meditation:** Mindfulness practices (discussed in more detail later in this chapter), such as meditation and mindful breathing, can help promote emotional well-being. These practices encourage staying present in the moment, reducing anxiety about the future or dwelling on the past (Liu et al., 2023).

8. **Hobbies and activities:** Engage in activities and hobbies that bring joy and a sense of fulfillment. Whether it's reading, gardening, painting, or any other passion, dedicating time to activities you enjoy can be a positive distraction and contribute to mental well-being.

9. **Hormone replacement therapy (HRT):** For some women, hormone replacement therapy (HRT) may be recommended to manage menopausal symptoms, including those affecting mental health. HRT can help balance hormonal levels and alleviate symptoms like mood swings and irritability. However, the decision to pursue HRT should be made based on your health history and considerations.

10. **Educate yourself:** Knowledge about the menopausal transition and its impact on mental health can empower you to navigate this phase with greater understanding.

11. **Limit caffeine and alcohol:** Although a steaming cup of coffee or a glass of wine can make you feel better, stimulants such as caffeine and alcohol can affect your sleep and exacerbate symptoms like hot flashes.

12. **Regular health checkups:** Regular health checkups with healthcare professionals can ensure that any underlying physical health concerns are addressed promptly. Physical health and mental health are closely connected, and addressing physical well-being can positively affect mental well-being.

It's important to recognize that each woman's experience of menopause is unique, and what works for one person may not work for another. Experimenting with different strategies and finding a combination that suits your individual needs is key. It is important to consult your doctor if mental health challenges persist or worsen. Overall, a holistic approach that combines physical, emotional, and social well-being is often the most effective way to support mental health during the menopausal transition.

Mindfulness and Meditation Techniques

Between work, children, aging parents, your significant other, and your home, women in their forties and fifties are juggling many balls with very little time left to take a moment for themselves. Practicing mindfulness techniques encourages you to turn your attention inwards and let go of your responsibilities, developing a new self-perspective. It means being one hundred percent present in the moment and allowing thoughts to pass through your mind without judgement, thus, promoting better emotional regulation and reducing stress (Liu et al., 2023).

Mindfulness and meditation techniques can, therefore, be valuable tools to help women navigate the physical and emotional changes that come with the menopausal transition. These practices can promote a sense of calm, enhance self-awareness, and provide effective coping mechanisms. Below are some mindfulness and meditation techniques that may be beneficial during menopause:

Mindful Breathing:

- Find a quiet and comfortable place to sit or lie down.

- Sit comfortably and close your eyes. Take a deep breath in, using your diaphragm to inhale the air deep into your lungs. Slowly exhale.

- Focus your attention on your breath, feeling the sensations of each inhalation and exhalation as your chest rises and falls.

- Don't worry if your mind wanders – it is normal. Gently redirect your focus back to your breath.

- Practice deep, slow breaths to help calm the nervous system and reduce stress.

Body Scan Meditation:

- Lie down in a comfortable position.

- Slowly scan your body by bringing your attention to each part in turn. Begin with your toes and gradually move up to the top of your head.

- Notice any sensations, tension, or areas of discomfort without judgment.

- While focusing on these sensations, breathe into the areas of tension, allowing them to release with each exhale.

Loving-Kindness Meditation:

- Sit comfortably and close your eyes.

- Begin by directing feelings of love and compassion towards yourself. Repeat phrases such as "May I be happy, may I be healthy, may I be at ease."

- Next, extend these wishes to others, starting with your loved ones and gradually expanding to include all beings.

- This practice can foster self-compassion and a positive emotional state.

Guided Imagery:

- Close your eyes and imagine a peaceful and serene place, such as a beach, forest, or meadow.

- Engage your senses by imagining the colors, sounds, and scents of this place.

- Spend a few moments immersing yourself in this calming mental environment.

Mindful Walking:

- Take a slow and deliberate walk, paying attention to each step and the sensations as your feet touch the ground with each step.

- Focus on your breathing, feeling the sensations as you inhale and exhale.

- Notice your surroundings - the colors, sounds, and textures around you.

- Walking mindfully can help ground you in the present moment and alleviate stress.

Mindful Eating:

- Practice mindfulness during meals by paying attention to the flavors, textures, and smells of your food.

- Eat slowly and savor each bite, being fully present in the act of eating.

- This practice can enhance the enjoyment of meals and promote mindful nourishment.

Mindfulness-Based Stress Reduction (MBSR):

- Consider enrolling in a mindfulness-based stress reduction program, which typically includes a combination of meditation, mindful movement like yoga, and group discussions.

- MBSR programs are designed to teach practical mindfulness skills for managing stress and promoting well-being.

Mindfulness Apps and Resources:

- Explore mindfulness and meditation apps that offer guided sessions specifically tailored for menopausal women. Apps such as Headspace, Calm, or Insight Timer often have specific meditations addressing stress, sleep, and emotional well-being.

Consistency is key when practicing mindfulness and meditation. Even short, regular sessions can have a positive impact over time. These techniques can empower you during menopause by providing tools to help you manage stress, enhance your self-awareness, and promote a positive and resilient mindset. Take your time and experiment with a variety of techniques to find the practices that resonate most with you and incorporate them into your daily routine for optimal benefits.

Strategies to Accept and Love Your Changing Body

Accepting and loving your body as your hormone levels start to drop and your appearance and health begins to change is a journey involving embracing the changes and developing a positive relationship with yourself. Apart from mindfulness and meditation techniques, there are several other strategies you can use to navigate this process and learn to love and accept the new version of yourself.

First, be kind to yourself. Treat yourself with the same compassion you would your best friend. After all, your body is undergoing a variety of natural changes because of fluctuating hormone levels, and it is okay to feel a range of emotions as you learn to live in your new body.

As such, it is normal to have negative thoughts about your body during the menopausal transition. However, they are not helpful and may lead to the development of mood disorders. It is important to acknowledge these thoughts and then replace any critical self-talk with positive affirmations. Try focusing on the positive aspects of your body and the personal qualities you value most about yourself. Recognize and celebrate your strengths, talents, and accomplishments that extend beyond your physical appearance. In doing so, it may be useful to keep a gratitude journal. Make a note of everything you appreciate about your body. Think about how it allows you to move or be creative. Be grateful for nurturing relationships and how your body continues to carry you through life despite the turbulence of menopausal symptoms. Practicing gratitude can help shift your focus from the negative aspects of the midlife change to embracing this time of your life. It enables you to pay attention to the habits that promote overall health and well-being like eating a balanced diet and exercising regularly.

To further enhance your new positive attitude, surround yourself with encouraging influences. People who uplift and support you give you the confidence you need to embrace the wise woman within you. You may consider joining communities or support groups, in-person or online, where women share their experiences during menopause. Connecting with others who are navigating similar journeys can provide validation, encouragement, and a sense of community. Finally, if a negative body image affects your mental health, consider seeking support from a mental health professional, such as a therapist or counselor. Professional guidance can offer valuable tools and strategies for cultivating a positive body image.

The journey toward accepting your evolving body during menopause is unique, and it is okay to progress at your own pace. Embracing the changes, nurturing a positive mindset, and being kind to yourself are essential elements for promoting love and acceptance for your body during this transformative phase of life.

Cognitive Behavioral Therapy (CBT)

Cognitive-behavioral therapy (CBT) is a therapeutic approach that can be highly effective for women experiencing challenges during menopause, particularly in addressing emotional and cognitive aspects of this life stage. Also, research shows that CBT delivered by a healthcare professional can also be useful in modifying your perception of vasomotor symptoms such as hot flashes. This type of therapy focuses on identifying and changing negative thought patterns and behaviors, promoting healthier coping mechanisms, and enhancing overall mental well-being (Hunter & Chilcot, 2021).

CBT can be beneficial for women during menopause in the following ways:

1. CBT helps women recognize and modify negative thought patterns associated with mood swings and anxiety during menopause. By challenging and changing distorted thinking, women can develop healthier responses to emotional fluctuations.

2. Sleep disturbances are common during menopause. CBT for insomnia (CBT-I) is a specialized form of CBT that focuses on improving sleep by addressing thoughts, behaviors, and environmental factors that contribute to insomnia. This can be particularly helpful for women experiencing disrupted sleep patterns.

3. CBT can help women develop effective coping strategies for managing physical symptoms like hot flashes. Learning how to change the way you perceive the symptoms and discovering new ways to respond when they occur can reduce the stress and discomfort you feel when your body temperature rises.

4. The changes in your body shape during menopause, along with hot flashes and mood swings, may result in a negative self-image. CBT can help you overcome a negative body image and develop a more realistic and positive view of your body, supporting good self-esteem and body acceptance.

5. Menopause is a stressful time for many women. CBT teaches you effective stress management techniques, including problem-solving skills, time management, and relaxation exercises, to cope effectively with high-stress levels.

6. Cognitive changes, such as memory lapses and difficulties concentrating, can be a source of frustration. CBT interventions can help you adapt to these changes by enhancing brain health and improving overall cognitive function.

7. CBT encourages the adoption of healthy lifestyle changes, including regular exercise, balanced nutrition, and adequate sleep. These lifestyle modifications can positively impact both physical and mental well-being during menopause.

8. Menopause often coincides with significant life transitions, such as children leaving home or changes in career. CBT helps women navigate these transitions by addressing thoughts and beliefs related to identity, purpose, and life satisfaction.

9. CBT can enhance communication skills, aiding women in expressing their needs and concerns to partners, family, and healthcare professionals. Improved communication can foster understanding and support during the menopausal transition.

10. Mood disorders such as depression and anxiety are common during the menopausal transition. CBT is an evidence-based treatment for mental health issues and can be adapted to address depressive symptoms by targeting negative thought patterns and promoting positive behavioral changes.

While there are self-help options, such as apps available to guide you through the process of cognitive behavioral therapy, it is best to consult with a qualified mental health professional such as a psychologist or licensed therapist. They can offer expert advice and tailor therapeutic interventions to your unique needs and concerns. Cognitive behavioral therapy is a collaborative and goal-oriented form of therapy offering several benefits for women navigating midlife.

Ignoring Your Mental Health is not an Option

Between the urgent demands of your physical health and the never-ending responsibilities associated with the middle years of your life, your mental health may be forgotten. Nevertheless, managing stress and taking care of your moods and brain function is just as important as ensuring your cholesterol levels and blood pressure fall within the normal range.

It is not an indulgence to step away from the demands of your daily life and give yourself a moment to turn your attention inward to check in and see how you are doing. Just as you would phone a friend when she is going through a rough patch, learning to be kind to yourself and treat yourself with the same compassion can make it easier to cope with the stress of modern living.

From mindfulness and meditation to cognitive behavioral therapy, there are many options to help you manage your stress, improve your mood, and increase your self-esteem. Your body is changing inside and out as you move towards menopause, but that is not a reason to resent it and have a negative body image. You may not appear as youthful as you did in your thirties, and you may be developing lines around your eyes, but those lines tell the story of your life. They are a reflection of the wise woman you have become over the last four decades of your life.

CONCLUSION

It cannot be denied that menopause is a challenging phase in a woman's life. For many, it can feel like the end of your monthly menstrual cycle marks the end of your usefulness in society. However, other societies embrace menopausal women and respect the wisdom they have gained throughout their reproductive life, raising a family while meeting all their other responsibilities.

Menopause is a natural transition that usually occurs in your forties and fifties. It results from a drop in the female reproductive hormones estrogen and progesterone. Girls are born with several hundred thousand fluid-filled sacs containing eggs in their ovaries. From the beginning of your menstrual cycle during puberty, a few follicles mature every month, with only one being released for fertilization. This maturation process stimulates the release of estrogen, and after ovulation, the remaining tissue produces progesterone.

Although these hormones are critical for reproductive health, they also have a significant impact on the structure and function of your body. They are what makes you uniquely female by promoting the growth of breast tissue and strengthening your pelvic bones for childbirth. In addition, these biological messengers support your immune and nervous systems, promote heart health, and maintain a healthy metabolism.

That is the reason it may seem like your body has lost the plot when you enter perimenopause – the period leading up to menopause. Gradually, you begin to notice signs that things are not as they used to be. For starters, your internal thermostat seems to have broken, and hot flashes become a frequent battle. Your moods also become less reliable, and you become more irritable and suffer mood swings without any forewarning. Furthermore, your doctor is suddenly warning you about high cholesterol levels and a rise in your blood pressure.

However, you are now armed with information about what to do when your hormones start toying with your physical and mental health. By keeping track of your menstrual cycle and symptoms, you will be able to judge whether you are in pre-menopause, perimenopause, menopause, or post-menopause. This knowledge also enables you to have an informed conversation with your doctor, who may order a battery of blood tests to help determine your hormonal status and the impact your fluctuating hormones have on your health.

They can also guide you in making decisions about how to manage your menopause symptoms. They may suggest lifestyle changes, including eating a balanced diet that supports your body through "the change," as well as exercise and stress management techniques. They are also in the position to help you decide whether hormone replacement therapy is a good choice for you.

However, if you decide to manage your menopause, a healthy diet forms the basis of your health plan. Now, more than ever, your body is relying on you to provide essential nutrients to support your physical and mental health. From an adequate calcium intake to prevent bone loss to eating enough protein to maintain strong muscles and ensuring that you consume enough essential fatty acids to reduce inflammation and control cholesterol levels, your health begins on your plate. The best diet is one that provides all of the energy and nutrients your body requires. It includes foods from all food groups – carbohydrates, proteins, fats, fruits, vegetables, and dairy products. While there is room for variation, your diet must meet your basic requirements.

Middle-age spread is real. As your hormone levels drop, your body fat levels rise, especially around your belly. As tempting as it may be to try a strict diet to drop a few extra pounds, restricting your calorie intake or omitting an entire food group can do more harm than good. It may be more challenging to lose weight in midlife, but it is not impossible. By eating foods that support your health and metabolism, you may also be able to prevent weight gain.

Of course, regular physical activity goes hand in hand with a healthy diet for health and weight loss. Not only does moving your body keep your heart in tip-top shape, but it also creates an energy deficit that can promote weight loss and help you maintain your weight. It is also critical for good mental health as it forces you to take your mind off your daily troubles and focus on breathing and putting one foot in front of the other. In addition, it promotes the release of feel-good neurotransmitters that give your mood a boost, even when you are feeling low.

That is something that happens to up to 64% of women during perimenopause. Your mood is affected by your declining hormone levels because they are involved in the production of neurotransmitters such as serotonin and dopamine, which help regulate your mood. As hormone levels drop, levels of these brain chemicals may also drop, resulting in mood swings, depression, and anxiety.

Therefore, it is crucial for overall health to learn how to support your mental health during menopause. Not only is the risk of mood issues higher at this time of your life, but your changing body may lead to you having a negative body image and poor self-esteem. Mindfulness meditation and other stress management techniques, along with strategies for shifting your focus to the positive aspects of your body and your life, can make it easier to cope with the ups and downs of the menopause transition.

Remember that you are not alone in your journey. All women undergo similar changes, and healthcare professionals, from your general practitioner to your gynecologist and your therapist, can help you navigate this significant life stage.

Educate yourself to remove the mystery that surrounds menopause and recognize this change as a gateway to your "wise woman status." After all, your body has undergone several transformations. The first was from being a girl into a young woman. Next, you may have embraced the miracle of childbirth. And now, you and your body have earned the respect of your community. It is time to be kind to yourself and embrace the wise woman within.

Afterword

If you've journeyed with me to the final page, thank you for your time and companionship along the way! Your readership is greatly appreciated, and it would be wonderful to hear your thoughts.

If you could spare a few moments to leave a review, it would not only help me to improve the storytelling but also assist fellow readers in finding their next great read.

Whether it's a few words of feedback or a detailed critique, all of your insights are invaluable. Thank you once again for choosing my book, and I hope to see you on the pages of one of my other books.

Warm regards,

Carina

REFERENCES

About Adult BMI | Healthy Weight, Nutrition, and Physical Activity | CDC. (2022, June 3). Centers for Disease Control and Prevention. https://www.cdc.gov/healthyweight/assessing/bmi/adult_bmi/index.html

Al-Atif, H. (2022). Collagen Supplements for Aging and Wrinkles: A Paradigm Shift in the Field of Dermatology and Cosmetics. *Dermatology Practical & Conceptual*, e2022018. https://doi.org/10.5826/dpc.1201a18

Alcohol & Menopause, Menopause Information & Articles | The North American Menopause Society, NAMS. (n.d.). North American Menopause Society (NAMS) - Focused on Providing Physicians, Practitioners & Women Menopause Information, Help & Treatment Insights. Retrieved October 27, 2023, from https://www.menopause.org/for-women/menopauseflashes/exercise-and-diet/drink-to-your-health-at-menopause-or-not

Barnard, N. D., Kahleova, H., Holtz, D. N., del Aguila, F., Neola, M., Crosby, L. M., & Holubkov, R. (2021). The Women's Study for the Alleviation of Vasomotor Symptoms (WAVS): a randomized, controlled trial of a plant-based diet and whole soybeans for postmenopausal women. *Menopause, 10,* 1150–1156. https://doi.org/10.1097/gme.0000000000001812

Batch, J. T., Lamsal, S. P., Adkins, M., Sultan, S., & Ramirez, M. N. (2020). Advantages and Disadvantages of the Ketogenic Diet: A Review Article. *Cureus.* https://doi.org/10.7759/cureus.9639

Bermingham, K. M., Linenberg, I., Hall, W. L., Kadé, K., Franks, P. W., Davies, R., Wolf, J., Hadjigeorgiou, G., Asnicar, F., Segata, N., Manson, J. E., Newson, L. R., Delahanty, L. M., Ordovas, J. M., Chan, A. T., Spector, T. D., Valdes, A. M., & Berry, S. E. (2022). Menopause is associated with postprandial metabolism, metabolic health and lifestyle: The ZOE PREDICT study. *EBioMedicine*, 104303. https://doi.org/10.1016/j.ebiom.2022.104303

Black Cohosh - Health Professional Fact Sheet. (n.d.). Office of Dietary Supplements (ODS). Retrieved November 29, 2023, from https://ods.od.nih.gov/fac tsheets/BlackCohosh-HealthProfessional/

Bleibel, B. (n.d.). *Vaginal Atrophy - StatPearls - NCBI Bookshelf.* National Center for Biotechnology Information. Retrieved November 22, 2023, from https://w ww.ncbi.nlm.nih.gov/books/NBK559297/

Bone Density Scan: MedlinePlus Medical Test. (n.d.). MedlinePlus - Health Information from the National Library of Medicine. Retrieved November 30, 2023, from https://medlineplus.gov/lab-tests/bone-density-scan/

BOUTAS, I., KONTOGEORGI, A., DIMITRAKAKIS, C., & KALANTARIDOU, S. N. (2022). Soy Isoflavones and Breast Cancer Risk: A Meta-analysis. *In Vivo*, *2*, 556–562. https://doi.org/10.21873/invivo.12737

Brooks, N. A., Wilcox, G., Walker, K. Z., Ashton, J. F., Cox, M. B., & Stojanovska, L. (2008). Beneficial effects of Lepidium meyenii (Maca) on psychological symptoms and measures of sexual dysfunction in postmenopausal women are not related to estrogen or androgen content. *Menopause*, *6*, 1157–1162. https://doi.org/10.1097/gme.0b013e3181732953

Cable, J. K. (n.d.). *Physiology, Progesterone - StatPearls - NCBI Bookshelf.* National Center for Biotechnology Information. Retrieved November 12, 2023, from https://www.ncbi.nlm.nih.gov/books/NBK558960/#:~:text=Progestero ne%20is%20primarily%20known%20as,plays%20a%20role%20in%20the

Calcium content of common foods | International Osteoporosis Foundation. (n.d.). International Osteoporosis Foundation | IOF. Retrieved October 26, 2023, from https://www.osteoporosis.foundation/patients/prevention/calcium-cont ent-of-common-foods

Cardwell, G., Bornman, J., James, A., & Black, L. (2018). A Review of Mushrooms as a Potential Source of Dietary Vitamin D. *Nutrients*, *10*, 1498. https://doi.org/10.3390/nu10101498

Casteel, C. O. (n.d.). *Physiology, Gonadotropin-Releasing Hormone - StatPearls - NCBI Bookshelf.* National Center for Biotechnology Information. Retrieved November 12, 2023, from https://www.ncbi.nlm.nih.gov/books/NBK558992/#:~:text=Gonadotropin% 2Dreleasing%20hormone%20(GnRH)%20is%20a%20crucial%20substance%20i n,sex%20hormones%20by%20the%20gonads.

Cena, H., & Calder, P. C. (2020). Defining a Healthy Diet: Evidence for the Role of Contemporary Dietary Patterns in Health and Disease. *Nutrients*, *2*, 334. https://doi.org/10.3390/nu12020334

Chen, Q., Wang, H., Wang, G., Zhao, J., Chen, H., Lu, X., & Chen, W. (2022). Lactic Acid Bacteria: A Promising Tool for Menopausal Health Management in Women. *Nutrients*, *21*, 4466. https://doi.org/10.3390/nu14214466

Ciappolino, V., Mazzocchi, A., Enrico, P., Syrén, M.-L., Delvecchio, G., Agostoni, C., & Brambilla, P. (2018). N-3 Polyunsatured Fatty Acids in Menopausal Transition: A Systematic Review of Depressive and Cognitive Disorders with Accompanying Vasomotor Symptoms. *International Journal of Molecular Sciences*, *7*, 1849. https://doi.org/10.3390/ijms19071849

Cienfuegos, S., Corapi, S., Gabel, K., Ezpeleta, M., Kalam, F., Lin, S., Pavlou, V., & Varady, K. A. (2022). Effect of Intermittent Fasting on Reproductive Hormone Levels in Females and Males: A Review of Human Trials. *Nutrients*, *11*, 2343. https://doi.org/10.3390/nu14112343

Conde, D. M., Verdade, R. C., Valadares, A. L. R., Mella, L. F. B., Pedro, A. O., & Costa-Paiva, L. (2021). Menopause and cognitive impairment: A narrative review of current knowledge. *World Journal of Psychiatry*, *8*, 412–428. https://doi.org/10.5498/wjp.v11.i8.412

Constitution of the World Health Organization. (n.d.). World Health Organization (WHO). Retrieved December 20, 2023, from https://www.who.int/about/accountability/governance/constitution

Delgado, B. J. (n.d.). *Estrogen - StatPearls - NCBI Bookshelf*. National Center for Biotechnology Information. Retrieved November 12, 2023, from https://www.ncbi.nlm.nih.gov/books/NBK538260/#:~:text=Estrogen%20is%20a%20steroid%20hormone,managing%20symptoms%20associated%20with%20menopause.

Dempsey, M., Rockwell, M. S., & Wentz, L. M. (2023). The influence of dietary and supplemental omega-3 fatty acids on the omega-3 index: A scoping review. *Frontiers in Nutrition*. https://doi.org/10.3389/fnut.2023.1072653

Desmawati, D., & Sulastri, D. (2019). Phytoestrogens and Their Health Effect. *Open Access Macedonian Journal of Medical Sciences*, *3*, 495–499. https://doi.org/10.3889/oamjms.2019.086

Dietary Guidelines for Americans, 2020-2025 and Online Materials | Dietary Guidelines for Americans. (n.d.). Home | Dietary Guidelines for Americans. Retrieved October 26, 2023, from https://www.dietaryguidelines.gov/resources/2020-2025-dietary-guidelines-online-materials

Elshaikh, A. O., Shah, L., Joy Mathew, C., Lee, R., Jose, M. T., & Cancarevic, I. (2020). Influence of Vitamin K on Bone Mineral Density and Osteoporosis. *Cureus*. https://doi.org/10.7759/cureus.10816

Faubion, S. S., Sood, R., Thielen, J. M., & Shuster, L. T. (2015). Caffeine and menopausal symptoms. *Menopause, 2*, 155–158. https://doi.org/10.1097/gme.0000000000000301

Feduniw, S., Korczyńska, L., Górski, K., Zgliczyńska, M., Bączkowska, M., Byrczak, M., Kociuba, J., Ali, M., & Ciebiera, M. (2022). The Effect of Vitamin E Supplementation in Postmenopausal Women—A Systematic Review. *Nutrients, 1*, 160. https://doi.org/10.3390/nu15010160

Follicle-Stimulating Hormone - Health Encyclopedia - University of Rochester Medical Center. (n.d.). University of Rochester Medical Center | UR Medicine. Retrieved November 30, 2023, from https://www.urmc.rochester.edu/encyclopedia/content.aspx?contenttyp eid=167&contentid=follicle_stimulating_hormone

Gietka-Czernel, M. (2017). The thyroid gland in postmenopausal women: physiology and diseases. *Menopausal Review*, 33–37. https://doi.org/10.5114/pm.2 017.68588

Hall, L., Callister, L. C., Berry, J. A., & Matsumura, G. (2007). Meanings of Menopause. *Journal of Holistic Nursing, 2*, 106–118. https://doi.org/10.1177/ 0898010107299432

Harper-Harrison, G. (n.d.). *Hormone Replacement Therapy - StatPearls - NCBI Bookshelf*. National Center for Biotechnology Information. Retrieved November 23, 2023, from https://www.ncbi.nlm.nih.gov/books/NBK493191/

Harvie, M., & Howell, A. (2017). Potential Benefits and Harms of Intermittent Energy Restriction and Intermittent Fasting Amongst Obese, Overweight and Normal Weight Subjects—A Narrative Review of Human and Animal Evidence. *Behavioral Sciences, 4*, 4. https://doi.org/10.3390/bs7010004

Health Effects of Overweight and Obesity | Healthy Weight, Nutrition, and Physical Activity | CDC. (2022, September 24). Centers for Disease Control and Prevention. https://www.cdc.gov/healthyweight/effects/index.html

Health screenings for women ages 40 to 64: MedlinePlus Medical Encyclopedia. (n.d.). MedlinePlus - Health Information from the National Library of Medicine. Retrieved November 30, 2023, from https://medlineplus.gov/ency/article/007 467.htm

Herbal Medicine | Johns Hopkins Medicine. (2021, September 24). Johns Hopkins Medicine, Based in Baltimore, Maryland. https://www.hopkinsmedicine.o rg/health/wellness-and-prevention/herbal-medicine

Hickey, M., Ambekar, M., & Hammond, I. (2009). Should the ovaries be removed or retained at the time of hysterectomy for benign disease? *Human Reproduction Update, 2*, 131–141. https://doi.org/10.1093/humupd/dmp037

Hormones | Endocrine Glands | MedlinePlus. (n.d.). MedlinePlus - Health Information from the National Library of Medicine. Retrieved November 12, 2023, from https://medlineplus.gov/hormones.html

How Does Social Connectedness Affect Health? | CDC. (2023, May 8). Centers for Disease Control and Prevention. https://www.cdc.gov/emotional-wellbeing/so cial-connectedness/affect-health.htm

Hoyt, L. T., & Falconi, A. M. (2015). Puberty and perimenopause: Reproductive transitions and their implications for women's health. *Social Science & Medicine*, 103–112. https://doi.org/10.1016/j.socscimed.2015.03.031

Hunter, M. S., & Chilcot, J. (2021). Is cognitive behaviour therapy an effective option for women who have troublesome menopausal symptoms? *British Journal of Health Psychology, 3*, 697–708. https://doi.org/10.1111/bjhp.12543

Hypothyroidism (Underactive Thyroid) - NIDDK. (2022, November 15). National Institute of Diabetes and Digestive and Kidney Diseases; NIDDK - National Institute of Diabetes and Digestive and Kidney Diseases. https://www.niddk.nih.gov/health-information/endocrine-diseases/hypothyroi dism#:~:text=Trials%20for%20Hypothyroidism-,What%20is%20hypothyroidis m%3F,the%20front%20of%20your%20neck.

Jin, J. (2017). Vaginal and Urinary Symptoms of Menopause. *JAMA, 13*, 1388. https://doi.org/10.1001/jama.2017.0833

Johnson, A., Roberts, L., & Elkins, G. (2019). Complementary and Alternative Medicine for Menopause. *Journal of Evidence-Based Integrative Medicine*, 2515690X1982938. https://doi.org/10.1177/2515690x19829380

Jordan, S., Tung, N., Casanova-Acebes, M., Chang, C., Cantoni, C., Zhang, D., Wirtz, T. H., Naik, S., Rose, S. A., Brocker, C. N., Gainullina, A., Hornburg, D., Horng, S., Maier, B. B., Cravedi, P., LeRoith, D., Gonzalez, F. J., Meissner, F., Ochando, J., ... Merad, M. (2019). Dietary Intake Regulates the Circulating Inflammatory Monocyte Pool. *Cell, 5*, 1102-1114.e17. https://doi.org/10.1016 /j.cell.2019.07.050

Katz, D. L., & Meller, S. (2014). Can We Say What Diet Is Best for Health? *Annual Review of Public Health*, *1*, 83–103. https://doi.org/10.1146/annurev-publhealth-032013-182351

Lephart, E. D., & Naftolin, F. (2022). Factors Influencing Skin Aging and the Important Role of Estrogens and Selective Estrogen Receptor Modulators (SERMs). *Clinical, Cosmetic and Investigational Dermatology*, 1695–1709. https://doi.org/10.2147/ccid.s333663

Li, T., Xiao, X., Zhang, J., Zhu, Y., Hu, Y., Zang, J., Lu, K., Yang, T., Ge, H., Peng, X., Lan, D., & Liu, L. (2014). Age and sex differences in vascular responsiveness in healthy and trauma patients: contribution of estrogen receptor-mediated Rho kinase and PKC pathways. *American Journal of Physiology-Heart and Circulatory Physiology*, *8*, H1105–H1115. https://doi.org/10.1152/ajpheart.00645.2013

Lin, S., Lima Oliveira, M., Gabel, K., Kalam, F., Cienfuegos, S., Ezpeleta, M., Bhutani, S., & Varady, K. A. (2021). Does the weight loss efficacy of alternate day fasting differ according to sex and menopausal status? *Nutrition, Metabolism and Cardiovascular Diseases*, *2*, 641–649. https://doi.org/10.1016/j.numecd.2020.10.018

Liu, H., Cai, K., Wang, J., & Zhang, H. (2023). The effects of mindfulness-based interventions on anxiety, depression, stress, and mindfulness in menopausal women: A systematic review and meta-analysis. *Frontiers in Public Health*. https://doi.org/10.3389/fpubh.2022.1045642

López-Pérez, M. P., Afanador-Restrepo, D. F., Rivas-Campo, Y., Hita-Contreras, F., Carcelén-Fraile, M. del C., Castellote-Caballero, Y., Rodríguez-López, C., & Aibar-Almazán, A. (2023). Pelvic Floor Muscle Exercises as a Treatment for Urinary Incontinence in Postmenopausal Women: A Systematic Review of Randomized Controlled Trials. *Healthcare*, *2*, 216. https://doi.org/10.3390/healthcare11020216

Luteinizing Hormone (Blood) - Health Encyclopedia - University of Rochester Medical Center. (n.d.). University of Rochester Medical Center | UR Medicine. Retrieved November 30, 2023, from https://www.urmc.rochester.edu/encyclopedia/content.aspx?ContentTypeID=167&ContentID=luteinizing_hormone_blood#:~:text=Men%3A%201.24%20to%207.8%20IU,0.61%20to%2016.3%20IU%2FmL

Maca: MedlinePlus Supplements. (n.d.). MedlinePlus - Health Information from the National Library of Medicine. Retrieved November 30, 2023, from https://medlineplus.gov/druginfo/natural/555.html#:~:text=Special%20precautions%20%26%20warnings%3A&text=Hormone%2Dsensitive%20conditions%20such%20as,do%20not%20use%20these%20extracts.

Magnesium - Health Professional Fact Sheet. (n.d.). Office of Dietary Supplements (ODS). Retrieved November 23, 2023, from https://ods.od.nih.gov/fac tsheets/Magnesium-HealthProfessional/

McCarthy, M., & Raval, A. P. (2020). The peri-menopause in a woman's life: a systemic inflammatory phase that enables later neurodegenerative disease. *Journal of Neuroinflammation, 1.* https://doi.org/10.1186/s12974-020-01998-9

Mentella, Scaldaferri, Ricci, Gasbarrini, & Miggiano. (2019). Cancer and Mediterranean Diet: A Review. *Nutrients, 9,* 2059. https://doi.org/10.3390/n u11092059

Miller, V. M., & Duckles, S. P. (2008). Vascular Actions of Estrogens: Functional Implications. *Pharmacological Reviews, 2,* 210–241. https://doi.org/10.1124/p r.107.08002

&NA; (2001). The role of calcium in peri-and postmenopausal women: consensus opinion of The North American Menopause Society. *Menopause, 2,* 84–95. https://doi.org/10.1097/00042192-200103000-00003

Nagy, B., Szekeres-Barthó, J., Kovács, G. L., Sulyok, E., Farkas, B., Várnagy, Á., Vértes, V., Kovács, K., & Bódis, J. (2021). Key to Life: Physiological Role and Clinical Implications of Progesterone. *International Journal of Molecular Sciences, 20,* 11039. https://doi.org/10.3390/ijms222011039

Nair, PradeepM. K., & Khawale, P. (2016). Role of therapeutic fasting in women's health: An overview. *Journal of Mid-Life Health, 2,* 61. https://doi.or g/10.4103/0976-7800.185325

Nedresky, D. (n.d.). *Physiology, Luteinizing Hormone - StatPearls - NCBI Bookshelf.* National Center for Biotechnology Information. Retrieved November 12, 2023, from https://www.ncbi.nlm.nih.gov/books/NBK539692/

Normal Thyroid Hormone Levels - Endocrine Surgery | UCLA Health. (n.d.). UCLA Health: Center for High Quality Health Care Services. Retrieved November 30, 2023, from https://www.uclahealth.org/medical-services/surgery/endocrine-surgery/conditi ons-treated/thyroid/normal-thyroid-hormone-levels#:~:text=TSH%20normal% 20values%20are%200.5,0.7%20to%201.9ng%2FdL.

Nowosad, K., & Sujka, M. (2021). Effect of Various Types of Intermittent Fasting (IF) on Weight Loss and Improvement of Diabetic Parameters in Human. *Current Nutrition Reports, 2,* 146–154. https://doi.org/10.1007/s13668-021-0035 3-5

Okeke, T., Anyaehie, U., & Ezenyeaku, C. (2013). Premature Menopause. *Annals of Medical and Health Sciences Research*, *1*, 90. https://doi.org/10.4103/2141-9248.109458

Oliveira, L. da C., Morais, G. P., Ropelle, E. R., de Moura, L. P., Cintra, D. E., Pauli, J. R., de Freitas, E. C., Rorato, R., & da Silva, A. S. R. (2022). Using Intermittent Fasting as a Non-pharmacological Strategy to Alleviate Obesity-Induced Hypothalamic Molecular Pathway Disruption. *Frontiers in Nutrition*. https://doi.org/10.3389/fnut.2022.858320

Orlowski, M. (n.d.). *Physiology, Follicle Stimulating Hormone - StatPearls - NCBI Bookshelf*. National Center for Biotechnology Information. Retrieved November 12, 2023, from https://www.ncbi.nlm.nih.gov/books/NBK535442/#:~:text=Follicle%2Dstimulating%20hormone%20(FSH),in%20both%20males%20and%20females.

Park, S., Kang, S., & Lee, W. J. (2021). Menopause, Ultraviolet Exposure, and Low Water Intake Potentially Interact with the Genetic Variants Related to Collagen Metabolism Involved in Skin Wrinkle Risk in Middle-Aged Women. *International Journal of Environmental Research and Public Health*, *4*, 2044. https://doi.org/10.3390/ijerph18042044

Patel, S., Homaei, A., Raju, A. B., & Meher, B. R. (2018). Estrogen: The necessary evil for human health, and ways to tame it. *Biomedicine & Pharmacotherapy*, 403–411. https://doi.org/10.1016/j.biopha.2018.03.078

Pavlović, J. M. (2020). The impact of midlife on migraine in women: summary of current views. *Women's Midlife Health*, *1*. https://doi.org/10.1186/s40695-020-00059-8

Peters, B., Santoro, N., Kaplan, R., & Qi, Q. (2022). Spotlight on the Gut Microbiome in Menopause: Current Insights. *International Journal of Women's Health*, 1059–1072. https://doi.org/10.2147/ijwh.s340491

Peycheva, D., Sullivan, A., Hardy, R., Bryson, A., Conti, G., & Ploubidis, G. (2022). Risk factors for natural menopause before the age of 45: evidence from two British population-based birth cohort studies. *BMC Women's Health*, *1*. https://doi.org/10.1186/s12905-022-02021-4

Porri, D., Biesalski, H. K., Limitone, A., Bertuzzo, L., & Cena, H. (2021). Effect of magnesium supplementation on women's health and well-being. *NFS Journal*, 30–36. https://doi.org/10.1016/j.nfs.2021.03.003

Purohit, P., Sassarini, J., & Lumsden, M. A. (2019). Management of Induced Menopause in Gynaecological Cancers and Their Challenges. *Current Obstetrics and Gynecology Reports*, *3*, 94–102. https://doi.org/10.1007/s13669-019-0262-x

Ranjan, P., Chopra, S., Sharma, K. A., Malhotra, A., Vikram, NavalK., & Kumari, A. (2019). Weight management module for perimenopausal women: A practical guide for gynecologists. *Journal of Mid-Life Health*, 4, 165. https://doi.org/10.4103/jmh.jmh_155_19

Rapkin, A. J. (2007). Vasomotor symptoms in menopause: physiologic condition and central nervous system approaches to treatment. *American Journal of Obstetrics and Gynecology*, 2, 97–106. https://doi.org/10.1016/j.ajog.2006.05.056

Rondanelli, M., Faliva, M. A., Tartara, A., Gasparri, C., Perna, S., Infantino, V., Riva, A., Petrangolini, G., & Peroni, G. (2021). An update on magnesium and bone health. *BioMetals*, 4, 715–736. https://doi.org/10.1007/s10534-021-00305-0

Ryczkowska, K., Adach, W., Janikowski, K., Banach, M., & Bielecka-Dabrowa, A. (2022). Menopause and women's cardiovascular health: is it really an obvious relationship? *Archives of Medical Science*, 2, 458–466. https://doi.org/10.5114/aoms/157308

Rzepecki, A. K., Murase, J. E., Juran, R., Fabi, S. G., & McLellan, B. N. (2019). Estrogen-deficient skin: The role of topical therapy. *International Journal of Women's Dermatology*, 2, 85–90. https://doi.org/10.1016/j.ijwd.2019.01.001

Santoro, N. (2016). Perimenopause: From Research to Practice. *Journal of Women's Health*, 4, 332–339. https://doi.org/10.1089/jwh.2015.5556

Santoro, N., & Randolph, J. F. (2011). Reproductive Hormones and the Menopause Transition. *Obstetrics and Gynecology Clinics of North America*, 3, 455–466. https://doi.org/10.1016/j.ogc.2011.05.004

Scott, A. J., Webb, T. L., Martyn-St James, M., Rowse, G., & Weich, S. (2021). Improving sleep quality leads to better mental health: A meta-analysis of randomised controlled trials. *Sleep Medicine Reviews*, 101556. https://doi.org/10.1016/j.smrv.2021.101556

Scott, A., & Newson, L. (2020). Should we be prescribing testosterone to perimenopausal and menopausal women? A guide to prescribing testosterone for women in primary care. *British Journal of General Practice*, 693, 203–204. https://doi.org/10.3399/bjgp20x709265

Shabkhizan, R., Haiaty, S., Moslehian, M. S., Bazmani, A., Sadeghsoltani, F., Saghaei Bagheri, H., Rahbarghazi, R., & Sakhinia, E. (2023). The Beneficial and Adverse Effects of Autophagic Response to Caloric Restriction and Fasting. *Advances in Nutrition*, 5, 1211–1225. https://doi.org/10.1016/j.advnut.2023.07.006

Smith, P. J., & Merwin, R. M. (2021). The Role of Exercise in Management of Mental Health Disorders: An Integrative Review. *Annual Review of Medicine, 1*, 45–62. https://doi.org/10.1146/annurev-med-060619-022943

Soare, A., Del Toro, R., Khazrai, Y. M., Di Mauro, A., Fallucca, S., Angeletti, S., Skrami, E., Gesuita, R., Tuccinardi, D., Manfrini, S., Fallucca, F., Pianesi, M., & Pozzilli, P. (2016). A 6-month follow-up study of the randomized controlled Ma-Pi macrobiotic dietary intervention (MADIAB trial) in type 2 diabetes. *Nutrition & Diabetes, 8*, e222–e222. https://doi.org/10.1038/nutd.2016.29

Sozen, T., Ozisik, L., & Calik Basaran, N. (2017). An overview and management of osteoporosis. *European Journal of Rheumatology, 1*, 46–56. https://doi.org/10.5152/eurjrheum.2016.048

Stanczyk, F. Z., & Clarke, N. J. (2014). Measurement of Estradiol—Challenges Ahead. *The Journal of Clinical Endocrinology & Metabolism, 1*, 56–58. https://doi.org/10.1210/jc.2013-2905

The American Heart Association Diet and Lifestyle Recommendations. (2021, November). The American Heart Association. https://www.heart.org/en/healthy-living/healthy-eating/eat-smart/nutrition-basics/aha-diet-and-lifestyle-recommendations

Thyroid and menopause article. (n.d.). British Thyroid Foundation. Retrieved November 22, 2023, from https://www.btf-thyroid.org/thyroid-and-menopause-article#:~:text=Women%20with%20pre%2Dexisting%20hypothyroidism,available%20to%20do%20its%20job.

Torres, S. J., & Nowson, C. A. (2012). A moderate-sodium DASH-type diet improves mood in postmenopausal women. *Nutrition, 9*, 896–900. https://doi.org/10.1016/j.nut.2011.11.029

USDA MyPlate What Is MyPlate? (n.d.). MyPlate | U.S. Department of Agriculture. Retrieved October 26, 2023, from https://www.myplate.gov/eat-healthy/what-is-myplate

Valdes, A. M., Walter, J., Segal, E., & Spector, T. D. (2018). Role of the gut microbiota in nutrition and health. *BMJ*, k2179. https://doi.org/10.1136/bmj.k2179

Vasim, I., Majeed, C. N., & DeBoer, M. D. (2022). Intermittent Fasting and Metabolic Health. *Nutrients, 3*, 631. https://doi.org/10.3390/nu14030631

Vetrani, C., Barrea, L., Rispoli, R., Verde, L., De Alteriis, G., Docimo, A., Auriemma, R. S., Colao, A., Savastano, S., & Muscogiuri, G. (2022). Mediterranean Diet: What Are the Consequences for Menopause? *Frontiers in Endocrinology.* https://doi.org/10.3389/fendo.2022.886824

Vincent, C., Bodnaruc, A. M., Prud'homme, D., Olson, V., & Giroux, I. (2023). Associations between menopause and body image: A systematic review. *Women's Health*. https://doi.org/10.1177/17455057231209536

Vitamin D | International Osteoporosis Foundation. (n.d.). International Osteoporosis Foundation | IOF. Retrieved October 26, 2023, from https://www.ost eoporosis.foundation/patients/prevention/vitamin-d

What Is Menopause? | National Institute on Aging. (n.d.). National Institute on Aging; https://www.facebook.com/NIHAging/. Retrieved November 13, 2023, from https://www.nia.nih.gov/health/what-menopause

Worthen, M. (n.d.). *Stress Management - StatPearls - NCBI Bookshelf*. National Center for Biotechnology Information. Retrieved December 20, 2023, from ht tps://www.ncbi.nlm.nih.gov/books/NBK513300/

Zouboulis, C. C., Blume-Peytavi, U., Kosmadaki, M., Roó, E., Vexiau-Robert, D., Kerob, D., & Goldstein, S. R. (2022). Skin, hair and beyond: the impact of menopause. *Climacteric*, 5, 434–442. https://doi.org/10.1080/13697137.2022 .2050206

Made in the USA
Las Vegas, NV
11 March 2024

87074395R00066